T0354332

'Madame,
may I have this
dance?'

ST. MARSEILLE, FRANCINE

'Madame, may I have this dance?'

'Self help'

TRAFFORD Publishing

Order this book online at www.trafford.com
or email orders@trafford.com

Most Trafford titles are also available at major online book retailers.

Note for Librarians: A cataloguing record for this book is available from Library
and Archives Canada at www.collectionscanada.ca/amicus/index-e.html

Printed in Victoria, BC, Canada.

ISBN: 978-1-4269-1606-9

*Our mission is to efficiently provide the world's finest, most comprehensive book publishing
service, enabling every author to experience success. To find out how to publish your book, your
way, and have it available worldwide, visit us online at www.trafford.com*

Trafford rev. 10/1/09

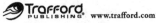 www.trafford.com

North America & international
toll-free: 1 888 232 4444 (USA & Canada)
phone: 250 383 6864 ♦ fax: 812 355 4082

I dedicate this book to all the people who helped me through this period in my life.

To each and every one of you, my most sincere THANK YOU!

I

The deception...

After having had René-Luc as a friend since I was nine years old and as my husband for over 24 years, all of a sudden one sunny Saturday afternoon, everything collapses. I find myself alone; he is gone! Why? He does not say! It is like that! I cry, I choke and I hurt so badly!

One night, as I am walking home from work, I see a middle-aged couple holding hands across the street. They stop for an instant and kiss.

As I stand there looking at them, my eyes fill with tears and I say to myself:
'This will never happen to me again!'

I cannot help thinking that MY LIFE is over! It is incredible; I am only 45 years old! What will become of me?

I put all the strength and the energy I have left into my work.

As we so often say:
'Time heals!'

7

After two years of solitude, the girls at the office invite me to celebrate the anniversary of one of the secretaries.

We laugh and have a lot of fun! From then on, I begin a new life; the adventure, the unknown...

Several years go by during which I have made new friends! One evening with a couple of girls from the office, we go to a dance Hall that is mostly for singles. Needless to say that I had never gone out dancing alone before! To my surprise, I find it very nice and I have a good time without spending the whole night drooling all over myself. For a couple of hours, I almost forget my pain!

This outing made me aware that I am not the only human being alone on this earth! It is incredible to see the number of lonely people around us! This wakes me up and I realize that life is too beautiful not to be lived to the fullest! I am feeling alive again!

It is in this same dance Hall called: 'Le Rendez-vous' that one Sunday evening, January 5th, 1992, while my friend Andrée and I are sitting there; all of a sudden a man tapes on my shoulder and asks:
"Madame, may I have this dance?"

As I turn to see who it is, to my amazement, it is the man I have been longing to dance with for quite a while. I had even talked to Andrée about him.

Very calmly, I say:

"I would love to, Monsieur!"

The feeling I have dancing this first Viennese waltz with him is very special! I have the impression that I am flying on a cloud! It is exactly the way I had imagined it all along!

Because it is winter and that I really hate to drive in winter, Andrée always picks me up and drives me back.

At this time, Andrée and I go dancing once a week and this is quite convenient for both of us. Of course, my dancing friend, whose name by the way is 'Peter', is always there and we dance together most of the time. We laugh and have a great deal of fun!

One night, while Peter and I are on the dance floor, Andrée joins us and says:
"I am very sorry but I really feel bad and I want to go home. I know it is early but honestly, I am not well at all!"

It is only 8H30, but since I came with her, I must go back with her; especially that she is not feeling well.

Peter, who heard our conversation, says:
"I will gladly drive you home if you accept to stay; it is still very early! Will you stay?"

I look at him and ask:
"Where do you live?"
"I live in the west end of town. Why do you ask this question?"
"That is completely out of your way; I live in the east end of town! You would have to make quite a detour!"

"I would even drive you to Three Rivers if it allowed us a few more hours of dancing and fun! Do not worry; I promise to drive you home! Will you stay?"

After all, Three Rivers is only about 200 km from here... We both burst out laughing and I gladly accept!

I tell Andrée that Peter offered to take me home and I make sure that she is well enough to get home safely. We both go back on the dance floor and enjoy ourselves until closing.

As promised, he brings me home, stops in front of my apartment, waits until I am inside and leaves.

What a gentleman! What chivalry! But most of all, what a wonderful evening! I had so much fun! I must admit that it has been quite a while since I have felt so good!

With time, a beautiful friendship develops between us! It soon becomes obvious that, seeing one another only once a week is not sufficient.

One night Peter asks me:
"Could you come dancing more often than once a week? We see one another only on Sunday! Can you come next Friday night?"
"Honestly, I do not like to go out alone! I cannot picture myself sitting at the end of a table waiting for an invitation to dance."
"If this is the only reason that stops you, I will sit with you and we will dance together all evening. Shall I see you on Friday?"

We end up meeting, at 'Le Rendez-vous' four nights a week! It appears that my desire to see him seems greater than my fear of driving in winter!

With time our feelings become more and more serious and one night, all of a sudden and without even looking at me, Peter asks:
"Are you a good 'cordon blue'?"

Stunned by the abruptness of the question, I look at him laughingly and say:
"My dear friend, I honestly have to admit that I am a big zero in the kitchen. I even succeed in burning boiling water..."

Approximately one month later, he looks at me and says:
"Would you mind very much to see someone else in your kitchen?"
"Actually, I would not mind at all! I am never there anyway!"

I had no idea how he would react to such an answer, but in all honesty, I had to tell him the truth.

It is true; I really do not like cooking and I am not good at it either! I love to do many different things, but cooking is absolutely not one of them!

A little while later, I look at him and very seriously, I say:
"You know, Peter, what you see is what you get. That is it..."

With a smile, he replies:
"The same goes for you my Dear!"

11

One evening Peter calls and asks if I am going dancing tonight! I can barely speak; I have a terrible cold. He says:
"I can hardly hear you, what is wrong with your voice?"
"I am sorry Peter, but I cannot go dancing tonight; I have a very bad cold and on top of it all, I am losing my voice."
"Do not worry a thing about it, I will bring you some of my chicken soup and it will cure you very fast."
"But Peter, you cannot be serious! There is a big snowstorm outside, or have you not noticed? You cannot cross the city simply to deliver a thermos of hot chicken soup!"

The first thing I know, the doorbell rings and he walks in with a big thermos. I could not believe he came all this way in such a storm! He pours a full cup and tells me to drink it while it is hot. The soup is delicious and soothing for my throat. After, he says:
"Now wrap yourself up in all the blankets that you have and sleep. You will feel a lot better tomorrow! I will call you in the morning!"

And he leaves.

On his way home that night, he realizes that his *'goose is cooked'*...

I slept like a baby and the next morning I felt better and my voice was back. I drank the rest of the soup and went right back to bed.

The following day, I felt well enough to return to the office.

A week later, I call my Father and ask him if I could come over for a visit. I would like him to meet Peter! The following Sunday, Peter and I go for a visit with my Father.

Peter and my Dad get along quite nicely and we have a good time. Once we are ready to leave, Peter and my Father shake hands and Peter walks towards the elevator while I kiss my Dad and say goodbye.

Once my Dad and I are alone, he whispers:
"He seems like a good man, but you know my daughter, he will never be a Frenchman!"

I have to tell you that my Dad is already 88 years old; a whole different generation! Nevertheless, I am very happy that he thinks that Peter is a good man!

I join Peter at the elevator and off we go dancing! What a wonderful day!

II

A new start...

From that moment on, Peter becomes more and more protective of me! He starts driving me back and forth to work every day.

Because it is only a seven minute drive from his place to my work, he suggests that I spend the week at his apartment (which we nicknamed: our summer residence) and we spend the weekends at my place (nicknamed: our winter residence).

Slowly Peter encourages me to start bringing some work-clothes such as; dresses, a few skirts, blouses and other essentials. In the meantime, he transfers his shirts, trousers and suits into a smaller closet.

The first thing we realize, his closet is filled up with my clothes while his clothes are all crushed in the small closet in the hallway.

One evening, as we are both at the 'summer residence', Peter looks at me for a while and says:

14

"What would you say if we were to move in with one another? During the week, we stay in the west-end because it is closer to your work and furthermore, I work downstairs. We go to your apartment only on weekends! Also very important, we would only have one rent to pay! I think it would be a good idea to find a bigger place not too far from here. It would be good for both of us!"

"Well, I cannot move in here with you, your place is too small and of course, you cannot move in with me; it is too far from our work!"

Finally, we both agree that it makes a lot of sense; we absolutely need to find a new place in the vicinity.

One night Peter wakes me up at 4 o'clock in the morning and tells me he had a dream. He starts recounting:

"In my dream, I saw a washroom with a Jacuzzi, a vanity with two sinks all burgundy and the floor and the walls were all covered in little squares of white and light pink ceramics. It was so pretty!"

As I am a visual person, I can just imagine it... That same morning, he calls me at work and says:

"Cookie, I met the janitor and he tells me that there is a four and a half room apartment to rent in the building. He nicknamed it: 'Le Cadillac' because it is very nice! He also said that if we are interested, we could visit it tomorrow night. What do you think of that?"

15

"It sounds interesting! Why wait until tomorrow night, ask him if it is possible to see it tonight?"

That same evening, we visit the apartment. As we enter, Peter says:
"Close your eyes Darling, I will guide you."

Once we stop, he says:
"Now, open your eyes!"

Believe it or not, there it was in front of my eyes! Exactly the same washroom he had described at four o'clock this morning. I could not believe it!

That is really too much! I look at him and say:
"You did see this apartment before!"
"No honestly, I have never seen it! I was not even aware that there was such an apartment to rent in this building!"

It is totally awesome and we also like the other rooms in the apartment very much. The janitor tells us:
"The owner of the block made several renovations and he and his family lived here one year before buying a new house. No one has ever lived in this apartment since."
"Are you saying that it is available now?"
"Yes, that is exactly what I am saying."
"How much is the rent?"
"$700.00 a month, hot water included."

Peter and I sign a two-year lease that same evening and key in hand, we return to the apartment to exam it more thoroughly.

The laboratory kitchen is so cute! The living room/dining room area is an open space and it is very big. There are two bedrooms; exactly what we need. The master bedroom has a huge closet and there is a lot of storage space. We really love it!

Every morning before moving in, Peter and I run down in our bathrobes with our towels and take a nice Jacuzzi. After that, we rush back upstairs and get ready to go to work. We are like two kids...

January 23rd, 1993, one year and 18 days after the famous:
'Madame, may I have this dance?'
we move into our new apartment. Lily, Marc-André, Eric and Rick are there to help us. They place all the big furniture in their respective places and put up the bed.

That same night, Peter and I sleep in our new apartment and are happy to have taken the decision to move in together. What a good feeling!

Several years ago, I thought my life was finished! Now, I found a new love, a nice apartment close to our work and to top it all, we are both very happy.

It goes without saying that we never know what tomorrow holds! Even if we have the impression that all the doors are closing around us; never forget that somewhere, a window opens!

During the four years that we live in this apartment, Peter and I often consider buying a condominium. Of course, we are very happy here and we like it very much; but we really want a place of our own!

One evening, while taking a nice long walk, we stop at the Pharmacy. Peter opens the door and walks in with me. Suddenly, without saying a word, he turns around and goes back in the entrance. He joins me holding a real-estate booklet in his hand.

Once we get back home, we open the magazine and start looking for our dream home. We circle condominiums that seem interesting to us!

The next day, I make a few appointments and we start visiting the following night. The second condominium that we see; it is love at first sight! We are overwhelmed and decide to make an offer.

On our way back home, we cannot stop talking about what we have seen and we review everything that pleased us in that condominium. Two days later, we call the real-estate agent and make him an offer. We give him 48 hours for an answer and specify that this is a final offer.

We still have several visits scheduled for the following night and although our minds are made up, we do have to respect our engagements towards the other real-estate agent.

Having found the condominium of our dreams, nothing else is interesting! We find faults everywhere!

On Wednesday, February 14th, 1996, 48 hours after making our offer, the real-estate agent calls and informs us that it has been accepted. What a wonderful gift for Valentine's Day!

The condominium is superb; the division is really to our liking. There are two bedrooms, which is exactly what we were looking for. The middle part is the living room/dining room area and it is very large. We are facing the waterfront and the whole facade of the condominium is covered with windows and patio doors. The living room patio door opens to one of the two balconies.

Adjoining the master bedroom, there is a big Jacuzzi; it is like an indoor pool... The other patio door is in the bedroom and it leads to the second balcony.

Even though we visited more than ten condominiums, we have never been shaken by any of them. The second condominium we saw really stayed in our minds and in our hearts!

When I return home from the office the following night, I see a huge bouquet of gorgeous red roses placed in the middle of the dining room table. I count 24 beautiful roses and each one is like porcelain. How nice of him to think of doing such a thing! I am so touched and appreciative!

The 30th of June 1996, moving time! Once again, the children are here to help us move into our new condominium.

Once everything is inside, Rick and Eric go out and return pushing a nice barbecue. Rick says:
"We all got together and thought this would please you both! With two balconies, it should be very useful! This is our 'welcome to your new condominium' present."

Peter and I are so touched and of course, very happy! Not only are they helping us move, on top of it all, offering us this wonderful gift... It is super!

We are very happy in our new home! Here we find peace and security!

As the saying goes:
'Nothing lasts forever!'

Six months after moving into our new condominium, we fall into a series of mishaps.

The Residence, where my Father is staying for over a year now, calls me at the office on Monday morning and informs me that my Father is not well and that I should come over as soon as possible.

I call Peter at work to tell him about the call I received and he says:
"Rick is here and he is leaving for the South Shore. I will ask him to pick you up at the office and take you to your Father. Courage my Darling, I will join you a little later!"

I received the call from the Residence on Monday and on Saturday December 7th, at 1H05 a.m., while Lily and I are by his side; my Father passes away!

No sooner I start getting over my Father's death, Lily calls to say:
"Mom, Marc-André was offered a two-year contract in Europe, close to Paris. We seriously talked it over, analyzed the pros and the cons and finally came to the conclusion that this could be a very good opportunity for all of us. Therefore, we decided to accept the offer! What do you think of that Mom? Is it not wonderful? I hope you are happy for us!"

I am flabbergasted, two years without seeing them, without seeing my 'Mine-Mines'! Two years is a very long time, but what can I say if that is what she wants. I take a deep breath and whisper:
"Yes Darling, it is wonderful and what a great experience for the 'Mine-Mines'! Do you have the date of the departure?"
"The children and I should leave during the month of July but Marc-André is scheduled to start his new job in two weeks. Thank God, we have two weeks; there is so much to do! We have to sell the house, divide our things between what goes to Europe or stays here in storage. All this in two small weeks! Marc-André will also be busy; he has to find a house, furnish it before we arrive, register the children at school and also learn a new job!"

"Of course Darling; I know exactly what you mean! You should remember when we left for Africa for three years! Your Father also had to leave before us and I was left alone to do the packing and the distribution and everything else. Four years after our return from Africa, we even went back for another four years. Do not worry too much Lily, Peter and I are here and we will do our utmost best to help you in every way we possibly can. You know you can count on us!"

Lily sells the house and has to move out for the beginning of May. So Cassandra, Karl-David and Lily come to live with us until their departure. We even registered Cassandra to the school close to our home so that she could at least finish her school year.

The five of us have wonderful moments all together. How nice it is to have them close to me like this!

I am still working, but when I come home at night, the table is set and the dinner is ready. We spend hours and hours talking and reminiscing; we do not want to lose one second and try to live every moment to the fullest! It is simply wonderful!

Needless to say, I take full advantage of their presence as I know that I will be a long time without seeing them. I think:
'I am very blessed to have them here with me for a couple of months and share these precious moments with them.'

22

One month before Lily and the children leave for Europe, my Sister-in-law calls and tells me that my Brother has cancer and is in a terminal phase.

Lily and the children take the plane on Tuesday, July 14th, my Brother is admitted to the Emergency Ward on Thursday, July 16th and on Saturday, July 18th at 4H00 a.m., the hospital calls and informs me that my Brother has passed away.

This is the drop that overflows the vase! I cannot make the difference between Lily and the 'Mine-Mines' gone overseas and my Brother's death.

The only thing in my mind is; they are all gone! It is too much for me to handle and I simply lose it.

Dancing becomes an effort! I have no breath, no resistance, I tire easily and I feel that my lungs are going to explode.

Peter does not understand what is happening to me; as a matter of fact, neither do I. Things get quite bad, I have no patience and he does not recognize me anymore!

We drift further and further apart and finally decide to put the condominium up for sale. We finally conclude that it would be best to separate! Yes, we have reached this stage; there does not seem to be any other way!

After over 50 visitors, not a single offer was made! It is unreal! This situation does not help my depressive system!

One night Peter says:

"Cookie, nothing happens for nothing in life! There has to be a logical explanation for what is happening to us now!"

Finally, a few months later and because we did not even receive one little offer, we take the condominium off the market.

Afterwards, Peter says:

"Darling, I have a confession to make; every time we leave the apartment, I touch my Ivory statue and tell her that we do not want to move from here. We are so comfortable on the waterfront! We have peace and quiet and most of all, we feel very secure in this building. Do you agree?"

I keep wondering: could it be because of the Ivory statue or more probably, because the good Lord himself has decided otherwise? I guess we will never know!

Whatever the reason may be, the fact is that we did not sell! After this, we never mention separation again! To the contrary, we become closer to one another.

With time, we realize that we have a lot more to give to each other and without a word; we make an unconditional U-turn! The love we share is very strong and we hang on to it with all our might.

Time goes by and I am always tired! I become more and more depressed and I still have this burn in my lungs. To say the truth, I honestly do not feel well at all!

While taking a shower one Saturday morning, I pass the washcloth on my right temple and suddenly I feel an acute pain. I also notice that it is quite swollen!

With everything that is happening and because my condition is not getting any better, Peter tells me:

"Cookie, I think that it is time that you call your family Doctor and take an appointment with her to find out what is really going on? I am sure she can prescribe a medication of some sort that could help you and make you feel better. You cannot go on like this much longer. What do you say?"

I know he is right and finally I call my Doctor and make an appointment.

When I see the Doctor, I tell her about the pain and swelling on my right temple and mention that I hit my head a few weeks ago and it made a big lump. It has been nearly three weeks and the lump is still there!

After a thorough examination, she says:

"I think we need to do a complete check-up to see what is actually going on. In the meantime, I will prescribe tranquillizers and give you the prescriptions for different exams. All you have to do is call for appointments. I will see you again once I receive all the results."

From then on, the roller-coaster begins!

One Doctor tells me:

"I only deal with serious cases! You should see a General Practitioner!"

Another one says:
"Your case is too serious for me; you have to see a Specialist in Plastic Surgery!"

The Plastic Surgeon coldly says:
"There is absolutely nothing wrong with your head, it is simply shaped like this!"

I am dumbfounded and angry by his clumsy and tactless answer. Abruptly, I say:
"I have never had lumps on my head since I was born! How can you say that my head is shaped like this, you are joking or what?"

Dazed by my answer and more so by the tone of my voice, he looks at me and without answering, he continues:
"On the other hand, I do not like the lump in your neck! I think it should be examined more closely because I do not find this normal at all. I want you to meet with a throat specialist, here in the hospital. Follow me to the reception desk and we will schedule an appointment for you, for tomorrow."

No sooner said, he walks out of the Ward and goes straight to the front desk where he tells the nurse to make an appointment for me tomorrow. Without even saying one word, the poor nurse takes an appointment slip, writes down the time and hands over the slip to the Doctor. He quickly takes a look at it and gives it to me!

The next day, the O.R.L. examines my neck, my ears and the inside of my mouth.

After the exam, he says:

"Your salivary gland could be blocked, it does happen some times. In order to make sure, I would like you to pass a scan and an ultrasound of the lump in your neck. I also recommend that a biopsy be made of the lump for analysis. The results should tell us more! In the meantime, here is a prescription for anti-inflammatory pills to help reduce the swelling. I will call you as soon as I receive the results."

Now begins a new chapter in our lives; the waiting, the worrying and the stress...

III

The waiting, the worrying, the stress...

Three months later, we still have no results from all the exams I have passed! It is very easy to say:

'No news is good news!'

That certainly is not enough for me! I have already passed all the required exams and I need to know what is going on. I think that it is a lot worse to sit here and wonder what is happening! The waiting is atrocious, it eats you up inside! I am going out of my mind!

The questions that go through my head are non stop and very scary! Notwithstanding the stress it causes to all of us!

I call my family Doctor and ask her what is going on? It has been three months since my last visit and I still have no results of all the exams I have passed. She replies:

"I have only received one result so far and I am waiting for the others to come in before I see you again."

I am so fed up of waiting and furthermore, I want results. I ask her:
"I still would like to see you! I cannot stand the wait any longer; it is intolerable! Could you please receive me tomorrow, if only to calm me down a little?"

She accepts to see me! Peter and I go to her office and while I am waiting in the exam room, I see that my file is open and I take a peek. On the first page, my eyes stop on the word 'metastasis'... My heart stops beating! My eyes get watery and my grey cells start running the big marathon!

Thousands of questions run through my mind and I do not know how to react! I scarcely hear the Doctor when she approaches and says:
"Given that you have been running from one doctor to another for over three months now, with hardly any results, I am going to call a research Specialist at the hospital and ask if she can see you as soon as possible."

Miraculously, the research Specialist answers! The Doctor gives her a few details of my case and asks her when she can see me.

When the Doctor comes back, she tells me that the research Specialist will receive me tomorrow morning.

She adds:
"Be sure to be at the hospital in the Emergency Ward for nine a.m.; the Specialist will meet you there!"

The next morning when Peter and I arrive at the hospital, we are taken in a little room to wait for the Doctor. When she arrives, she tells us right upfront:
"We are going to hospitalize you for a few days, (which actually turned out to be nearly two weeks). As your Doctor was explaining to me; it appears that you have been running from hospital to hospital for quite a while, which is unfortunate, and that you still have not received any or few results of your tests. By being hospitalized, it will be easier to make all the required tests thus give us a better chance to obtain results."

Peter and I are startled! I really did not expect to be kept in the hospital that quickly as, on top of it all, we are in the middle of December and Xmas is just around the corner. She notices our hesitation and says:
"Do you want to know what is wrong with you?"
"Of course we want to know what is wrong; we simply did not expect this!"

She leaves and a nurse comes in with a stretcher and rolls me to a mini private room. Peter returns home to prepare a little suitcase with a few necessities because I did not think of bringing anything with me!

Once in the room, I cancel all the other appointments that I had scheduled by saying that I have been hospitalized. I could not find a better reason to give them!

That same afternoon, the exams start: several blood tests, x rays of all kinds, ultrasounds, electrocardiograms, and more... This goes on for days: scans, one biopsy after another. More blood tests several times a day, more analysis, etc... Test after test after test; will it ever end?

Eight days later, I am still hospitalized and I still have no results! It really looks grim! I am very nervous and so are the children and Peter. What more can we do but sit tight, hope and pray for the best!

Finally, on Xmas Eve, one Doctor comes and signs my release from the hospital saying: "Not much goes on in the hospital during the Holiday Season! We will let you go home to celebrate Xmas with your family. Come back on the 27th of December and do not worry; we will keep the room for you."

Xmas this year is not appealing to none of us! To say the truth, no one is really in the mood for celebration.

Before I was hospitalized, Lily had invited both her family and Marc-André's family for Xmas Eve celebration. Of course there is no way we can desist ourselves now and besides, how could I do this to Cassandra and Karl-David, they are both still so young and so happy that I am finally out of the hospital. Xmas is such a big thing for them!

Peter and I get all dolled-up and off we go to celebrate Xmas Eve with our loved ones!

Needless to say that everyone is aware of the difficult period we are living right now. Fortunately, no one questions us and I am very thankful for that!

The atmosphere is very tense but we try our best to be merry and have fun! After a lavish meal, and because the children cannot wait any longer to open their gifts, we all gather around the Xmas tree. Lily, who plays 'Mama Clause', sits on the floor and distributes the presents; to the children first, of course...

At midnight, the phone rings and it is Marc-André's father who lives quite far. He is calling his children and grandchildren to wish them all a very Merry Xmas and the best for the Holiday Season.

After his call, Lily says:
"Well, I have a Father too!"

She picks-up the phone and calls him!

Once the children and grandchildren have talked with him, Lily takes the phone and comes towards me. She asks:
"Mom, would you consider talking to Daddy and wish him a Merry Xmas?"

Their Father and I have not spoken in over five years! Considering the present circumstances and feeling that all the eyes are on me, what else is there to say but:
"Yes of course Darling!"

She hands me the phone and I wish him a Merry Xmas. After offering me his best wishes, he says:

"The children keep me informed on your health condition and all that has happened in the past three months or so. Would you mind if I called you, once in a while, to see how you are?"

"Of course I do not mind! You can call whenever you want!"

After that call, Cassandra, comes towards me with tears in her eyes. She puts her arms around me and says:

"Thank you so much Mamie for accepting to talk with Pappy, you have no idea how happy you have made me."

Even though she is only eleven years old, my poor little Darling suffers from our separation.

This gives me a double reason to be proud of what I did; not only by accepting to talk with her Pappy but more so to have made them happy. Even Lily and Eric have tears in their eyes! The celebration continues with big smiles on all the faces!

In the car on the way home, Peter says:

"I am so proud of you Sweetheart! You have made a lot of people very happy this Xmas Eve. One day you will realize all the good that you did tonight..."

Time has proven him right!

IV

The diagnostic...

The morning scheduled for my return to the hospital, December the 27th, I receive a call from the hospital asking me to go to the O.R.L. Ward. There, I have to see the O.R.L. surgeon who performed the first biopsy on the right side of my neck.

When I get there, the Doctor says:
"I have good news and bad news!"

My God! The stress and the anguish I feel at this instant are indescribable! It really does not sound good! I am not reassured at all and yet, I look at the Doctor and risk asking him:
"What is the bad news Doctor?"
"In the different analysis, we diagnosed what we call in medical term; 'a non-Hodgkin lymphoma, great cells B, stage IV'."

Making an enormous effort not to burst out in tears, I ask the Doctor:
"In plain English Doctor, is it 'cancer'?"
"Yes unfortunately, it is!"

"Now tell me Doctor, after such an earthquake, what good news can there be?"

"The good news is that it can be cured with the right treatments!"

I have wanted to know for so long! Well, now I know and I wish I never did...

When I come out of the O.R.L., Peter comes towards me and asks anxiously:

"What did the Doctor say? Did he have any results to give you?"

I simply cannot talk! I am choking and I am afraid to burst out in tears in front of the people. I walk towards the exit and Peter follows me and waits patiently.

Finally, with the little strength I have left, I tell him what the Doctor told me. Of course, tears are running down our faces! I look in his eyes and try to seek answers to my numerous questions:

'What are we going to do? What is going to happen to me? Am I going to die? What will become of us?'

I need answers, I must decide now what I am going to do; let it be or fight it! I cannot leave the hospital without knowing what we are going to do! Dear God, please help us! What should we do?

There at that precise moment, the answer comes in a flash! We both take the important decision that we are going to fight this, fight it with all our strength and may the good Lord help us!

The hospital informs me on what has to be done! Most importantly: meet with an Oncologist as soon as possible, to talk about the kind of chemotherapy treatments that would be best for me; then get as much information as possible on this type of lymphoma and find everything we can that could help me fight this terrible sickness.

As soon as Peter and I arrive home, we have a good long cry and once we calm down, we start surfing on the Internet to find everything we can on this specific type of cancer. We read on the different stages of this sickness (stage IV is the highest). We look for medications that could help and every possible way to fight this awful disease.

Exactly twelve days after being diagnosed, on the 8th of January 2002, Eric, Peter and I meet the Oncologist that has been assigned to me. He flat out tells us:
"If you do not get chemotherapy treatments as soon as possible, your life expectancy could be reduced to a few months."

Thank God I am sitting down, I feel I am going to faint! Eric, Peter and I are chocked! We cannot believe what we have heard and yet, the Oncologist did say those exact words right there in front of us. I do not understand and I say to myself:
'What on earth did he say? 'Only a few months to live'! No, this is not possible! We must have misunderstood! This cannot be!'

Seeing our total disarray and after leaving us to our thoughts, the research Nurse, who is standing next to the Doctor, presents herself and gently says:
"I am a Protocol Research Nurse and I am working on a project dealing with your type of cancer. It would be good if you accepted to take part in this study. Here is a copy of the Protocol and you should read it very carefully. If you have any questions concerning the Protocol, I will be pleased to give you names of patients with whom you could discuss it."

We are like robots; we do not seem to be able to think straight! Our bodies are sitting there but it is as though our minds have deserted us! I think we understood what the Doctor said; only we absolutely do not want to believe it!

Finally, Eric takes the Protocol and glances through it. He looks at me and says:
"Mom, I think you should consider signing this Protocol. It will surely do you no harm!"

Without even reading it, I simply sign! I must admit that this is the best advice my son ever gave me. I have never regretted it; to the contrary, I have often felt privileged by it!

Given that Peter and I had decided to fight this sickness and after recovering our senses, I look at the Doctor and say:
"Tell me what to do and I will do whatever it takes! Dear Lord, please help me! I need You now more than ever!"

The Doctor asks the research nurse (whom I will call henceforth: my guardian Angel), to prepare the necessary forms for all the exams I have to pass before it can even be decided on which chemotherapy treatment would be best for me.

Two days after our visit to the Doctor's office, the tests begin: electrocardiograms, lung x rays, scans, ultrasounds, blood tests and much more...

The Saturday afternoon, before my first chemotherapy treatment, René-Luc calls:
"The children informed me of your recent visit with the Oncologist. I was terribly shocked listening to what they were saying! It is really hard to accept such disappointing news! When you feel up to it and if you agree, it would be nice if you and I could have lunch sometime."
"I guess it would be good to have a good talk about all this over lunch! The children must have mentioned that I will receive my first chemotherapy treatment this coming Tuesday. As I do not have the slightest idea of how I am going to react to it and if we do decide to meet, I think it would be best not to wait too long. I do not want to rush anything, but honestly, I have no idea of what is waiting for me. I hope that you understand my point of view!"
"I understand very well! Would you agree to make it for lunch tomorrow?"
"I think tomorrow is good! Call me to confirm and give me the time!"

René-Luc calls Sunday morning and picks me up at 11 o'clock.

Eric had often mentioned to Peter that he would like to see his parents on good speaking terms and that, one day, the four of us would get together for dinner.

At the restaurant, René-Luc tells me about Eric's wish to which I reply:
"I think it would be nice to get together with the children. But honestly, I prefer to wait and see how I will react to the treatments before deciding anything."
"There is absolutely no rush! Whenever you feel up to it then we will set a date."

We have a nice lunch and talk easily! No bad feelings whatsoever!

Fourteen days after meeting with the Oncologist, I receive my first chemotherapy treatment. I am so scared and so nervous! As a matter of fact, we all are! I had no idea what the side effects would be, nor how I would react. We hear so many negative side effects concerning chemotherapy...

During these 14 days, Peter never leaves my side. He drives me to the hospital at six a.m., waits for me day in, day out. Sometimes we spend the whole day in the hospital. He sits there and waits, never complains, always encourages me and gives me a lot of strength. Needless to say that sometimes, I feel like throwing everything overboard and stop it all! It is so terribly hard!

Lily, Eric and Rick often come by and spend some time with us. They invite us out for dinner, when I feel well! They truly do their utmost best to distract us as often as they can. In these trying times, we most certainly need all the distraction we can manage and we really appreciate their efforts! Believe me; this is very good for both our morals!

Of course, as we all know, chemotherapy treatments are very hard and have huge side effects; tiredness, loss of appetite, weakness and so much more...

Four days after my first chemotherapy treatment, Peter, who has been cooking for us since we are together, concocted a soup specifically for me. It contains a lot of iron, tons of vegetables of all sorts. We baptized it: the 'miracle soup'. He even blends it because at times, I cannot even chew my food! This way, all I have to do is drink it!

Whether it is the soup, the good luck, or both, during my six months of chemotherapy, I never had anemia once and this, to the great amazement of the Oncologist. Usually, when you receive chemotherapy, your red blood cells drop drastically. Thanks to the 'miracle soup', mine stayed normal. The white blood cells dropped to zero several times!

Peter always tells me:
"Cookie, if you do not eat properly, you will lose your strength and there is no way you will be able to fight back against this sickness."

Therefore, he makes sure that I eat and rest well. He wants to put all the chances on our side. He accompanies me to all the treatments and stays by my side the entire time. He comes to the hospital for every appointment, for every blood test and the numerous exams. He is totally there for me!

When people say that support of your surrounding is nearly 50% of the cure, I honestly can say that it is more like 75% for me. Quality support is the most important thing in a sickness like this. The comfort of their presence, the reassurance and the constant love that they all give me are very positive benefits that help me keep my sanity and give me the will to fight this monstrous atrocity. I can only thank You, Dear Lord, for placing each one on my road!

Peter's first wife had cancer and was sick for ten years. Although he had promised himself to never get involved in another similar situation, nevertheless he stands by me and does his utmost best to make things easier. His son Rick often tells him:
"Pop I am so proud of you for staying with her, for supporting her and for encouraging her the way you do! I want you to know that I am here for you whenever you need me!"

Exactly fourteen days after my first treatment, I start losing my hair! In order not to have the pain of seeing them fall in bunches, I ask Peter to shave my head.

What a shock when I see myself in the mirror for the first time! I cannot get over my baldhead! Even if Peter tells me that I have a very pretty round head, it does not make me feel any better! It takes a while to get use to it and to accept it! At the beginning, I always wear my wig or a scarf on my head, but with time, I start going around the house bareheaded. I say to myself:
'After all, this is not the end of the world; there are a lot worse things in life!'

One day, when the 'Mine-Mines' are here, I ask them if they want to see what their Mamie looks like with no hair? Of course, at first they say 'no thanks'! A few hours later, they both come towards me and ask me to take-off my scarf. At the beginning, they are both shocked, but with time they say that this new look is 'cool' and it suits me very well!

Two months after my first chemotherapy treatment and after taking my regular blood tests, my guardian Angel calls and says:
"The blood tests show that your white blood cells are very low and that you should be hospitalized and in isolation. Your antibodies are non-existent and you have absolutely no defense. Should you have the misfortune of catching a simple cold or the slightest virus, you could die from it!"

I find myself back in the hospital and in isolation! During these five days, I start receiving 'Neupogen' injections.

42

'Neupogen' injections force my bone marrow to reproduce new white blood cells and help me regain good defensive antibodies. I stay in the hospital for five days and during that time, I have lung x rays and several electrocardiograms. I must not forget the numerous blood tests that they take every day to make cultures.

Thank God, I am allowed to receive visitors, as long as they agree to wear the mask! René-Luc comes in the morning, Eric passes by around lunchtime, and Lily comes as often as she can. Peter usually arrives around five p.m. and spends the evening with me. I must say that I did not find my stay in the hospital too hard given that I had all my loved ones surrounding me!

When I return home, I am still very fragile and weak and I have to be extremely careful not to be exposed to sick people and not to go in public places. In other words, the best thing to do is stay home quietly, rest and recuperate my strength!

At times, I am more than one month without seeing my darling 'Mine-Mines'.

Children often pick-up viruses at school or from other kids and because of my constant low white blood cells, I cannot allow myself the risk of getting any kind of infection. I find this very hard not to be able to see them more often. When they are in top shape, they always take the time to come and see us.

No one ever said that cancer is easy, and I am far from saying it myself! On top of the pain, the numerous blood tests; the exams one after the other, I have to be deprived of my loved ones; this makes it so much more difficult!

No, I am far from saying that cancer is easy, to the contrary! Even though we go through several difficult episodes, we must never stop fighting, never stop hoping and never stop praying.

Since I was diagnosed, that famous day of December 27th, 2001, my priorities have changed completely. My main preoccupation now is to fight and fight some more! I realize that I have no time to waste; life can be very short sometimes!

I want to bite into life and live life to the fullest! I thank God for all the help He gives me every day. When I go to bed at night, I thank the Lord for the wonderful day He so generously gave me. I ask Him to please watch over my sleep hoping that He will give me another tomorrow!

My second stay in the hospital follows a visit with the Oncology specialist. When he checks my blood test results, my white blood cells are down to zero again. He sends me to the Emergency Ward and from there; I am taken to an isolation room.

Once again, Peter goes home to prepare my suitcase!

The first thing the nurses do at the hospital is: take several blood tests in order to make cultures. After that, they send me for a lung x ray, an electrocardiogram and more blood tests.

The following day of my admission, Lily comes to spend the day with me. She arrives with croissants and coffee and we have breakfast together.

She has to wear a mask; nevertheless we are so happy to be together! We are chatting when all of a sudden we hear voices rising at the nurse's desk. There is a woman standing next to the nurse and we can hear her say:
"..... he does not want to pass that test, he says it hurts too much and he does not want to go through with it."

Trying to calm the woman, the nurse replies:
"I will tell the Doctor to be careful when he passes the tube. I will tell him to go slowly!"
"You do not seem to understand; he does not want to pass this test."
"Are you telling me that he will refuse to pass the test when the Doctor arrives?"
"That is exactly what I am trying to make you understand!"

Lily and I look at one another and we are startled! We both think:
'Why bother coming to the hospital if you do not want to undergo the tests, have the exams and receive the treatments?'

The hospital is not an amusement park! You have sick people and a lot of pain and anguish here! When you are hospitalized, it is because you are sick and you need treatments! We need the hospital, not the contrary!

I learned a lesson that day; I promised myself that whatever they ask me to do, whatever they want to do to me, whatever is necessary, painful or super painful, I will not say 'NO' to any test or cut or anything else. I am here to be cured; I am fighting for MY LIFE and whatever it takes... Oh Lord, give me the strength! Please help me get through it all!

A few days after my second stay in the hospital, Lily calls and says:

"Mom, Cassandra's First Communion is scheduled for the month of May and she would really like both of you to be there. I do not have the exact date yet, but as soon as I have it, I will let you know immediately. You will come? She would be so disappointed if you were not there!"

"What a question Sweetheart, of course we will be happy to attend her First Communion. I hope to be in good shape! We certainly do not want to miss this event for anything!"

A week or so later Lily calls back and says:

"Mom, I finally have the date for Cassandra's First Communion. It will take place on Sunday, May 5th, 2002; I hope that you will both be able to attend!"

46

"Darling, I promise you, we will do our utmost best to be there! In fact, the only reason that could stop us from being present is if I am in the hospital! Otherwise, tell Cassandra to count on us."

After her call, a wonderful idea crosses my mind as to what would be a very special gift for Cassandra's First Communion! Without wasting one second, I call René-Luc and tell him about it. He also thinks it is a very good idea and says he will come over this weekend to organize everything.

The first gift René-Luc gave me when we started dating in 1961 was a crystal rosary. I thought that, if we have the rosary nicely polished and buy a little purse to put it in, Cassandra's First Communion would be the ideal occasion to give her such a present!

After all, we are her Grandparents and this crystal rosary would be a very nice souvenir from both of us!

As understood, Saturday morning René-Luc comes by and we talk about how we will proceed for this special event. He says he will have the rosary polished!

After discussing, René-Luc asks if I am strong enough to go to the shopping centre to buy the little purse for the rosary and look for a nice First Communion card for Cassandra.

When René-Luc returns with the polished rosary, we will compose a little text and include it in her card.

Finally May 5th and my white blood cells are doing well! Peter and I prepare to go to church for Cassandra's First Communion!

It is so nice to see all the children gathered around the altar as they hold hands and sing together! This is very emotional for me! I must say that whatever concerns my little Darlings always touches me deeply!

Cassandra is so pretty with her long blue skirt and her pretty blue top! She looks like a little princess!

After church, we all go to Lily and Marc-André's place to celebrate! Lily ordered a nice buffet and it is very good! René-Luc had a chef pastry cook make a special First Communion cake for Cassandra. Not only is it beautiful, it is also delicious!

What a glorious day we had! I thank God for giving me the strength to be part of this special occasion in Cassandra's little life. I really appreciate the time He gives me with my beloved children and grandchildren. Being with them is not only an extraordinary feeling, but there is no price to the great joy it gives me.

A few times during my chemotherapy, I felt chest pains and because of that, I had to undergo several electrocardiograms and so far, the results have returned negative. The Oncologist always asks questions about the condition of my heart. Two days after Cassandra's First Communion, I meet with the Oncologist and he says:

"Because you felt chest pains during your chemotherapy treatments, I would like you to go for another electrocardiogram and also an ultrasound test called: 'mibi persantin'. This is a special test for the heart that gives a better view of its condition. I also think you should meet with a Cardiologist. In the meantime, I will prescribe nitroglycerin pills and should you ever feel chest pains, simply put one pill under your tongue. The pain should go away in a few minutes! You will not receive your chemotherapy treatment this week; your white blood cells are still too low. The nurse will make all the appointments and will call you with the details. I will see you again once we receive all the tests!"

In all, I was hospitalized and kept in isolation three times during my chemotherapy treatments and all for the same reason: low white blood cells.

Every time I was hospitalized, René-Luc would come in the morning to warm up my 'miracle soup' and he always made sure that I drank it all before leaving.

Eric came around lunchtime! He often came in with a bag containing chicken breasts or club sandwiches, or whatever...

As for Lily, due to her numerous responsibilities and to the fact that she lives and works on the South shore, she came whenever possible. Peter spent the evenings with me! So far, he has never missed one!

It is always pleasant to see them all and it gives me so much strength, energy, love and willpower to continue fighting! What an extraordinary support team! I can only thank them, over and over, for all they do for me!

After a few days of rest, we get the 'Mine-Mines' to come over and spend a few days with us. The presence of my little Sweethearts does wonders for me!

Although I have to take it easy and rest, we still have a lot of fun! We go to the pool several times a day, we play cards and society games that they enjoy so much. The children set the table and wash the dishes. Peter prepares healthy meals that we all appreciate. We have such a super time!

One month after my last chemotherapy and after undergoing all the necessary control tests, my guardian Angel calls and says that the Doctor would like to see me. She schedules an appointment for two days later.

Lily, Eric, Peter and I meet at the hospital for my appointment. When we enter the Doctor's office, they both have huge smiles on their faces as they look at the delegation; we are four... We sit down and the Doctor says:
"Madame, the chemotherapy treatments seem to have done wonders for you and were a great success. All the exams are very good and we see no more sickness! Therefore, I am very proud and pleased to tell you today that you are in *'remission!'*"

We sit there and stare at him! No reaction whatsoever! After a few seconds, it starts to sink in and our faces illuminate like Christmas trees. (So they said afterwards).

'REMISSION'! What a lovely sound this word has after so many hardships! We laugh and cry tears of joy! We rejoice yet, through all this euphoria, we do not forget to thank the Dear Lord for giving me another chance to life and allowing us to live such happy moments together.

I write these lines with tears in my eyes! At the same time, I say to myself:
'Is it really true? Am I really in remission? I find it hard to believe, it seems so incredible and I am nearly afraid to believe it! It seems too good to be true! We see the Doctor sitting there, in front of us and he did say 'You are in 'REMISSION'!'

We left the 'Mine-Mines' with their Pappy, therefore we are very anxious to spread the good news! We are so excited to finally bring them such wonderful news!

As we arrive at René-Luc's, we start all over again, laughing, crying, rejoicing and just being very happy! René-Luc opens a bottle of champagne and, all together, we toast to my 'REMISSION'.

After such excitement, we all return home lighthearted and filled with happiness! The 'Mine-Mines' come back with us and spend the rest of the summer.

Each day is a gift and we enjoy ourselves immensely! To not have this horrible sickness hanging constantly over my head is fantastic! It gives me wings and we are all deliriously happy!

Less than one month after being told that I was in '*remission*' and having lived such ecstatic joy, I discover a lump on the back of my neck. I call my guardian Angel to tell her about it and she says:

"This is a psychological reaction and it is quite normal after all that you have been through. Enjoy yourself and stop looking for lumps!"

I know that she is right and I try to take her advice! I cannot help myself; I constantly touch the lump to see if it is growing or, if by miracle, it is going! Unfortunately, day after day, the lump is still there and this does not help my nervous system at all!

Thank God the 'Mines-Mines' are still with us! I do everything I can think of to keep them busy thus keeping me from always thinking of this horrible lump that keeps growing in my neck.

At the end of the summer vacation, Cassandra and Karl-David go back home and prepare for their return to school.

A few weeks later, the lump is still there and it has gotten bigger! I decide to call my guardian Angel again and seeing how worried I am, she thinks it would be best to advance my appointment with the Doctor.

One week later, I meet with the Doctor and he examines my neck immediately. Inevitably, he discovers the lump that is causing me so much pain! He seems really surprised!

He asks my guardian Angel to schedule a Gallium Scan, an electrocardiogram, several blood tests and a few more tests. He also asks her to call me back to schedule another meeting once the results are in.

Here we go again; the waiting, the worrying... Unfortunately, our euphoria did not have a very long life!

Nearly one month goes by and still no news! We are so anxious and so worried! Finally, when my guardian Angel calls, she tells me that the results are in and that the Oncologist would like to see me. She gives me an appointment for the following week.

When Peter and I arrive in the Oncologist's office, he says:
"The test results are back and there is a spot on the Gallium scan that you passed. It is a spot and we cannot say for sure if it is cancer or simply an infection. I think we need to undergo more tests to find out exactly what this really is!"

After having said this, he calls the Dermatologist and asks if she can see me today. At the same time, he asks her to examine the lump and see if she can make a biopsy and have it analyzed.

We see the Dermatologist and after examining the lump closely, she says:
"I cannot perform a biopsy on your neck; first because of the location of the lump and second because it is too deep. You need to see a Plastic Surgeon Specialist. He alone can perform this kind of biopsy."

The Dermatologist calls the Plastic Surgeon and schedules an appointment for me in two days.

Two days later, once again Peter and I are back to the hospital! We meet with the Plastic Surgeon and right there, in his little cubicle and without even an explanation, he performs the biopsy. Peter is awe-struck!

When the Surgeon injects the liquid for the local anesthesia, I honestly think I am going to die! To say that it is painful would be a huge understatement!

Peter simply stands there and holds my hand! Once the area is frozen, the Doctor makes the incision, cuts off a piece of the lump and sets it aside to be analyzed. He stitches the wound and acts as if all this is nothing!

Once I recollect myself, the nurse brings a wheelchair and Peter wheels me to the car and helps me in.

As soon as we arrive in the apartment, I go straight to bed! Peter gives me some painkillers to ease the pain. He tries to make me eat my soup, but it is no use! The pain gets worse as it unfreezes!

Once again, we have to wait for results! Waiting is such a terrible thing! It creates anguish and anxiety and it drives me crazy...

Three weeks later; still no results and the area that I was operated on is swelling again. It is also very painful! I do not understand what all this means nor what is going on! Is the lump coming back? It is growing very fast!

I call my guardian Angel to explain the situation. She can tell by my voice that I am anguished and she says that she will talk to the Doctor immediately.

She calls back and says:
"The Doctor will go and see the Pathologist to talk about the results of the analysis of your last biopsy and this new situation. I promise to call you as soon as I have some news!"

My guardian Angel calls the next day and schedules an appointment with the Oncologist for the following week.

Peter and I meet the Oncologist on Tuesday! He says:
"After discussing the subject with the Pathologist, there appears to be no lymphoma in the piece that was analyzed. On the other hand, we cannot be sure whether it is or not the sickness."

The Doctor examines the lump and notices that it is indeed growing. He asks my guardian Angel to make appointments for a Gallium scan and another biopsy to further pursue the investigation.

My guardian Angel schedules the required appointments and calls back with the details.

Early the next day and totally discouraged, I call my guardian Angel and say: "No need to continue making all the required appointments because I have just discovered another lump that is about one inch above the first one. It is also very painful!"

She calls the Oncologist, informs him of my new discovery and asks him if he still wants the scan and the biopsy!

The Doctor says:
"We will keep the Gallium Scan and wait for the results after which, we will have a better idea of what to do next."

The waiting is terrible, the uncertainty is terrible but when the Doctor himself does not seem to have answers for this bizarre new situation, then the questions flow:
'What is happening to me? Where do I stand now? What is going to happen next? Is the cancer taking over my body? Is it generalizing? Am I dying?'

All these questions roll in my mind and it simply will not stop spinning! To think that no later than one month ago, I was in 'remission', it is so unbelievable... I am so frightened! The queries build up so fast in my head and it is really scary at times. I have the impression that I am looking at a horror movie and believe me, I am scared stiff!

56

In the meantime, I get more and more severe headaches. They become more frequent and last longer from one time to the next.

Even though I take analgesics every four hours, then every three; nothing doing, they do not help at all! The pain does not go away! There are days when I can hardly get out of bed; the pain is that severe! I honestly do not know what to do anymore, where to turn...

After a few days and unable to stand the pain any longer, I decide to call my guardian Angel to tell her:
"I really feel very bad! I am sure that there is something terribly wrong! I cannot function any more! The pain is so severe that I am unable to stand or sit; I cannot support the weight of my head at all. I take pills every hour and they do nothing! I really do not know what else to do! I am totally exhausted! There is no way that I can go on like this; I am going out of my mind! If only you knew how painful it is! Please, do something, you must help me!"
"I will call the Doctor immediately! He will prescribe painkillers that should help calm the pain. I will get back to you shortly!"

Half an hour later, she calls and says:
"Given that your Doctor is not on standby this week, I have scheduled an appointment with the Oncologist that is on standby this week and he will examine the lump thoroughly and will surely prescribe stronger medications. That is sure to help!"

The following morning, Peter takes me to the hospital to see the other Doctor. She examines the lump carefully and is stunned to see how big it is. She prescribes strong painkillers to take every four hours.

On our way back from the hospital, Peter stops at the pharmacy to pick up the prescription and I start taking the pills immediately. Unfortunately, even the stronger painkillers have no effect! Peter is worried sick; he does not know what to do anymore!

After taking the prescription painkillers for two days and two nights, on top of the analgesic pills that I take every hour, I still feel no relief. I call my guardian Angel again:
"Nothing helps! The painkillers plus the other pills that I take every hour simply do not help! The pain is excruciating! I honestly do not know what to do anymore! If only you knew how much I am suffering! Can you please help me; I do not know how much longer my heart will endure this pain!"

She talks to the Doctor and he prescribes an in-between pill to take two hours after the stronger pill, plus the analgesic pills every hour. In all, I take an average of 35 pills per 24 hours and I still feel no relief. Peter calls me his 'two-legged drug store'!

I try putting a bag of ice on the lump, but I cannot stand the cubes, they hurt too much! I am unable to touch my head, the pain is so excruciating!

All of a sudden and without saying a word, Peter puts on his coat, goes out, and returns with a bucket full of snow.

He fills a 'Ziplock' bag with snow, punches the middle of the bag with his fist to make a round and gives it to me. I slowly put the bag on the lump. The round of his fist in the bag seems to hug the lump. About one hour or so later, I start feeling a little relief.

I think that the combination of the snow plus the huge quantity of medications that I take help sooth the pain a little bit. What a good idea! I am still incapable of sitting or standing! I still cannot support the weight of my head; the pain is intolerable!

I feel totally drugged with all the medications I take! I have a hard time pronouncing the words right! Several times, day and night, Peter goes out on the balcony and fills up a Ziplock bag with snow.

When my appointment date comes up to see the Doctor, I even go to the hospital with my bag of snow. I cannot go without it! It is as though the snow keeps the lump at a certain cold temperature and it eases the pain. As soon as the Doctor sees me in the doorway of his office, he says:

"What happened to your face, it is all swollen? I can hardly recognize you!"

"Doctor, I told you that the pain was extremely severe and that I could not stand nor sit very long because the pain becomes too unbearable."

Without even examining me, he takes me to a room, makes me lie down and says:
"I will hospitalize you immediately!"
"But why Doctor? The operation is in three days, why hospitalize me now?"
"I cannot let you leave the hospital with such pain! I really do not understand what can cause such an acute pain!"

After a while, an aide wheels me directly to the room without even going through the Emergency Ward. As soon as I arrive in the room, a technician enters and passes me an electrocardiogram.

The Doctor requires several tests and blood tests to be made before the operation. From then on, I receive intravenous painkillers every four hours. Sometimes I even find it impossible to hold out longer than three hours. The nurses also make sure that I constantly have my bag of crushed ice.

I do not remember ever having suffered to this extent in my entire life, not even when I gave birth to my children.

Lily and Eric are discouraged to see me in this condition. They all feel so helpless; they would so much like to take the pain away! Through it all, they never give up hope!

It becomes a real obsession for Peter that I pull through this! To this day, he always hopes that I will make it and this gives me more strength to continue fighting even harder. He always tells me:

"Sweetie, you have to continue to fight! You cannot give up now, not now that we have come so far!"

Finally, the morning of the operation arrives! Can you believe that I am very happy! I so want the pain to go away!

Once in the operating room, the Plastic Surgeon greets me by saying:
"You must not worry, this is a minor operation; 15 to 20 minutes to the most. Relax and everything will be fine!"

Eight hours later, I am still not back in the room. Lily, Eric and Peter are waiting and wondering what could have gone wrong? Unable to stand it any longer, Eric goes to the nurses' desk and asks what is delaying my return? What is taking so long?

One nurse tells him:
"There has been a little problem during the operation but everything is fine now! She should come up shortly."

Eric returns in the room and tells them what the nurse said. You can imagine their stress; they were already very worried!

Finally, an hour and a half later, I am taken back to my room still drowsy and very much in pain.

I know that the children and Peter are there! I do not have the strength to talk to them but I can feel that Peter is holding my hand and is trying to give me all the strength he possibly can. I can also hear Lily and Eric crying!

Very soon, a nurse comes in and injects me a sedative! It knocks me right out! When I come too, they are all still there and Lily says: "Mom, try not to worry, I will stay the night with you. If you need anything at all, I will be right here!"

I whisper:
"Sweetheart, go home and rest! The nurses will keep me asleep all night and I am sure that I will feel better in the morning!"

They all kiss me one after the other and, leave heartbroken!

The next morning, the Oncologist comes to see me and says:
"Now I understand why you were in such excruciating pain! When they performed the biopsy on the first lump, they cut a nerve and of course, with time, the nerve grew. When the lump came back and got bigger, the nerve grew inside the lump. Therefore, every time you moved your head, the nerve was compressed and this is what caused the unbearable pain. This is why the minor operation that the Surgeon predicted would last between 15 to 20 minutes became a major operation. When the Surgeon cut the lump, he realized that the nerve was attached to the lump. He had to do something; he could not simply cut it off! I have scheduled several tests for you before you leave the hospital. I want to keep you under observation a few days longer and make sure that everything goes well."

Approximately ten minutes after the Doctor leaves, Peter walks in holding a thermos of my 'miracle soup' and it is nice and hot. While I sip my soup, I tell him everything the Doctor told me! Now we both understand why I was in so much pain! It is so good to be able to sit up in bed and support my head without hurting so!

The nurse comes and makes me sit on the edge of the bed. She advises me not to stand up because I am not strong enough yet.

Fifteen minutes later, Lily comes in with Cassandra. Poor little Darling, she is all shaken to see me like this! She cuddles up close to me and does not move. It feels good to have her this close! I want to comfort her because it hurts me terribly to see her so sad and worried. I am very proud that she had the strength and the courage to come with her Mother. Karl-David is still too young and, on top of that, he does not like hospitals!

After they leave, our friends Andrée and Renald come for a short visit and Eric arrives with his girlfriend. Needless to say that the little room is completely full!

Peter is happy to see all these nice people around me. He knows that this is a very good therapy for me and most of all that it makes me extremely happy.

What a beautiful day! I am sitting in bed, my head is very straight and I hardly feel any pain. What a relief to be nearly pain free!

Too often, we take our bodies for granted, but when a part of our body does not function properly, we are stunned and yet it happens frequently. Thank you for this wonderful day Dear Lord!

The following days, they remove the big dressing and the drain. I am taken down for the stomach ultrasound and a Gallium scan. They also take several blood tests!

The last day, Eric comes and we have lunch together. The Doctor signs my release and Eric helps me gather my things. I call Peter and ask him to come and pick me up. How good it feels to go home!

A little more than one week after leaving the hospital, my guardian Angel calls and says: "The Doctor wants to see you tomorrow, after your visit with the Plastic Surgeon that did the operation."

We see the surgeon and he examines the wound. He is satisfied with the operation and finds that everything is good! After seeing him, we go up to the Oncology Ward to meet with the Oncologist.

IV

The big decision...

As soon as we enter the Doctor's office, I sense that something is wrong; the Doctor is not his usual self! He is very serious and does not even examine me as he normally does. He invites us to sit down and goes right to the point, saying:

"Unfortunately, the sickness has returned! The lump that the Surgeon operated on was full of lymphoma. After consulting with the Oncology team, we came to the conclusion that two options are available in this case:

- the first option: when you get a lump, we will treat it. If another lump appears, we will treat it again, and so on until there are no treatments left to be had. Your life expectancy would then be between 18 to 24 months;

- the second option, more drastic, consists of an auto graft of the bone marrow. The chances are: 40% total cure, 45% that the sickness will recur and 10 to 15% of chances of dying."

Peter and I sit there totally numb! Nothing comes out, we simply stare at the Doctor and I think to myself:
'What on earth is he saying? Back to 18 to 24 months to live! I absolutely do not want to hear this! This is not possible! There must be a mistake somewhere!'

The Doctor waits a few minutes; I guess he is giving us time to start breathing again! He continues saying:
"The second option is a lot more complicated! It is an auto graft of the bone marrow and consists in a full check-up before even being eligible for the auto graft. If all the tests are satisfactory, the following steps will be taken:

1. One day of strong chemotherapy treatment in order to bring your white blood cells down to zero;

2. 10 to 12 days of 'Neupogen' injections in your stomach to force your bone marrow to reproduce new white baby blood cells;

3. you will come to the hospital for three or four consecutive days to retrieve your baby blood cells that will then be sent to a special department to be frozen;

4. you will then have a period of two to three weeks to rest. After this rest you will be hospitalized for three to six weeks in isolation. Once hospitalized, you will receive five-full days of chemotherapy. This will kill your blood cells, including the platelets and also the bone marrow.

After two days of rest, the Oncologist will re-inject your previously collected frozen baby cells via transfusion. After, you will have a period of 10 to 12 days of 'Neupogen' injections to re-stimulate your bone marrow to create new red and white blood cells and your platelets. I have now given you a quick overview of an auto graft of the bone marrow!"

Peter and I are shattered. Tears roll down our cheeks! The Doctor looks at us, waits a while; nothing, absolutely nothing! Very gently he says:
"Why not go home and reflect on everything I have just said? Analyze the situation and call me in a few days to give me your answer."

Like a robot, I look at the Doctor and ask: "What do you think I should do? I do not know what to do; I am unable to think straight! Please Doctor; give me an idea of what would be best for me?"
"I am sorry Madame; this decision is not mine to make! With such a serious undertaking, this has to be your decision and yours alone. It is not for me to tell you what to do in this case; you really have to decide by yourself."

I look at Peter and he too is crying! I take his hand and ask him:
"What should we do Sweetie? I honestly have no idea! Please help me!"

He looks at me and in a murmur says:
"Do we really have a choice my Darling?"

At that precise moment, I remember the important decision we took when I was diagnosed on that famous December 27th, 2001 and all of a sudden, I know exactly what I want to do and what I am going to do! I look at the Doctor and say:

"Well Doctor, from the day I was diagnosed, we promised ourselves we would fight to the utmost. Here is my decision: we will take our chances with the second option and may the good Lord give us strength and courage!"

"That is fine! Although you must understand that: if at any time you want to change your mind, you have to let me know and we will stop the process. Do you understand, at any time! This is a very big undertaking and you have the right to change your mind!"

I simply nod and we leave.

Once at home, I through myself into Peter's arms and we cry like babies. I do not know how long we stood there! We sit on the sofa and the tears continue rolling down our faces! After a long while, we start talking about the whole thing, all that it involves. Believe me it is a huge handful!

Suddenly I realize that I did not call the children! To say the truth, I have no desire to call them at all! Because I gave my word to keep them informed on whatever happened I have to call them now! Peter and I decide that it would be best to talk with them alone and in person and I agree with him.

I call Eric and trying very hard not to burst in tears, ask him:

"Hello my Darling! Do you have anything on your agenda tonight?"

"Why are you asking me this Mom? What is wrong?"

"Sweetie, I need to talk to you and Lily together. Are you free tonight?"

"Whatever was on my agenda tonight is not important at all! What time do you need me to pick you up Mom?"

"Eric, I have to call Lily and make sure that she is available. She has children you know! I will call you back!"

"Do not worry Mom, I will call her and arrange everything and pick you up in half an hour, is that convenient for you?"

"Yes Darling, I will be ready!"

By the time we get to Lily's place, they both know that there is something very wrong for me to summon them like this.

The three of us sit in the living room and I start recounting what the Doctor told us. They listen carefully while I speak and tears roll down their cheeks. I would like to see myself trillions of miles away from here! The more I talk, the more they hurt! It is terrible! When I stop talking, they both ask:

"Mom, what on earth are you going to do?"

"I took my decision in the Doctor's office this morning: I have decided to go forward with the auto graft of the bone marrow!"

"But Mom, you are not serious! You cannot take such an important decision just like that! We need to talk about this! We have to reflect on all that is involved and weight the pros and the cons. You must take more time before taking such a big decision! Do you realize how serious and dangerous this is? We need to discuss the whole thing together. This is your life we are talking about! You cannot play with your life! You cannot expect us to agree just like that on such an importance matter... Mom, did you not think of us before making such a big commitment? And what about the 'Mine-Mines', did you not think of them? This is so serious; you must take more time to think about all this!"

As I listen to them, I know they are hurting badly! Of course, this is their Mother's life that we are talking about! At the same time, I realize that they do not agree with the decision I took.

After waiting a while, I continue saying: "My poor Sweethearts, I am very much aware of the seriousness of my decision! I find it very difficult to try to explain why I took such a decision. You must try to understand my point of view! I could not see myself leaving the Doctor's office without knowing what I was going to do. I simply cannot stand the unknown anymore! The constant waiting and the stress that all this causes all of us! I am at a stage where things have to be clear in my head.

I need to know what comes next! I absolutely must know! Can you understand that? I know how serious this is, I know that I am taking a big risk, I even know that my life is in danger and that I could die. But would you rather have me sit there and wait for the next lump, get treatments, lose my hair every time, go back home and wait for the next lump until there is no more treatments left to be had? Do you understand that my average span of life would be reduced to 18-24 months with this option? Would you prefer that for me? What about quality life? Have you thought about that? How could I live in constant wait of one lump to another, one treatment to another, one month to another? What kind of life would I have just sitting there waiting? You know me better than that! You know very well that I cannot live, day by day, without knowing, without hope! As I just said, I cannot live in waiting anymore; I need to know! I must take this risk! What else could I do? This seems to be the only avenue that I have left! At least, this option gives me a 40% chance of hope!"

"Mom, you know that we are here for you and with you and you also know that we will always support you whatever decision you take. We love you Mom, but we are so afraid... Can you understand that?"

"Yes I understand that and Peter and I are also very scared. But little hope is better than no hope at all, do you agree with me?"

"We understand Mom and we will not let you down; we will stay by your side all the way! You can count on our full support and our love. We love you so much Mom!"

We hang on to one another and have a good long cry. It helps a little! Suddenly the doorbell rings, the children are here! So, very quickly, Lily says:

"You know Mom, Cassandra is aware of everything that has happened to you since the beginning of your sickness. She asks questions and I answer! I think I should tell her what has happened today! Is this all right with you?"

"Do you really think it is necessary to tell her now? Could you not delay it for a while? I think you should take some time to digest all this! Are you not afraid that this will scare her more than anything else?"

"No Mom, if she hears about this elsewhere, she will be very hurt! I honestly think it is best to tell her now?"

What else can I say but:
"Mom knows best!"

We dry our tears and greet them with smiles on our faces...

When Karl-David sees our teary eyes, he zooms off to his room! Cassandra sits with us in the living room and very softly, choosing her words carefully, Lily tells her what is going on. Tears roll down her cheeks. I find this so hard! My poor little Darling, she is so young to have such great pain! My heart hurts so badly!

While I spend some time with Lily and Eric, Peter goes to see Rick to give him the latest news and take some energy from him. Rick listens closely and encourages him as much as he can. He says:
"Pop, do you realize how much she needs you now? You must stay strong and try to give her all the energy, the strength and the courage she needs especially with everything that she is going through. Do not forget Pop, I am right here with you and for you. You can call on me any time; I will give you all the support I can. Stay strong and keep the courage!"

Exactly five days after having taken my decision, the tests begin: Maxilla facial, respiratory functions, cardiac ultrasound, PET scan, biopsy of my right hip, isotopic ventricular, several blood tests, urine tests. Name them; I pass them all...

I have three, sometimes five tests per day whenever possible. Peter is always by my side! He drives me from one hospital to another, he sits and waits and counts the bricks on the wall. How patient can a human being be? If I go by Peter's patience, I guess we could simple say: 'it is unlimited'. I do not know many people who could endure and give so much of themselves day-in day-out!

We also have to attend several meetings pertaining to the auto graft of the bone marrow. First, we meet with a specialist and she informs us of every step along the way.

She hands us pamphlets on the subject and a cassette of an auto graft of the bone marrow from beginning to end. She strongly suggests that we view it several times and write down all the questions that come to mind. She schedules another meeting in two weeks. We come out of there totally bushed! Our heads and hands are full!

That following evening Peter and I decide to view the cassette. My good Lord, what an undertaking! This is huge! There are so many difficulties, severe infections, high fever... All the different stages I will be going through! It never stops! This is nothing to reassure neither one of us...

We note all our questions and are very anxious to get the answers! As the auto graft specialist suggested, we view the cassette several times and the questions multiply.

In the meantime, Peter and I decide to take full advantage of the free time that we have before the auto graft.

Saturday night, we decide to go dancing! Believe me, with all that is happening right now, we really need the distraction! Andrée and Renald are there and we talk a lot!

It has been quite a while since our last outing and several friends come over and tell us how happy they are to see us again. It really feels good to see everyone! We do not dance very much, but to our amazement, we have a very good time!

After having finished the required exams and once all the results are in, the Doctor calls and informs me that I am eligible for the auto graft of the bone marrow. Now, the big journey begins!

One morning while showering, I discover a lymph node in my neck! I call my guardian Angel who in turn calls the Doctor.

She calls back saying:
"Given that you will soon be receiving your first chemotherapy treatment in view of the collection of your baby blood cells, the Doctor suggests that you verify the progression of the lump closely and wait for the treatment."

The next morning, I feel a second lump under the first one! I am extremely nervous and anxious to get that famous chemotherapy treatment!

The sickness seems to be taking over and it is going very fast! Peter and I are totally stressed and nervous! The treatment should slow down the progression; at least this is what we are hoping and praying for!

Finally, I receive my first chemotherapy treatment. It lasts from eight a.m. to three p.m.

During this treatment, the Doctor comes by and asks Peter and me to follow him.

Oh no! Not more bad news! This is not happening! Unfortunately, it is!

The Doctor says:
"One of the numerous blood tests has detected Hepatitis, type B!"

"Hepatitis, this is impossible, how can this be? Where on earth could I have caught such a thing?"

Because of this new finding, everyone in my surrounding has to be tested: Lily, Eric, Peter and even René-Luc. Thank God, all the results returned negative!

Now we will have to add one more specialist to the already long list of Doctors: a Hepatitis specialist who inevitably will require more blood tests and more exams... It is as though when it starts, it never ends!

Because this new discovery concerns the liver, the Oncology specialists are very worried. They even ask themselves whether they will be able to go through with the auto graft of the bone marrow!

The Hepatitis could cause serious problems and bring serious complications! After worrying ourselves sick and nearly going out of our minds, the Doctor calls and says:

"We will go forward with the auto graft! It goes without saying that we will have to be very careful and take many more precautions. You will also have to take medications for a period of at least two years to make sure that the process of the auto graft will not have damaged your liver."

After the chemotherapy treatment, once again I begin the 'Neupogen' injections for nine consecutive days to force my bone marrow to reproduce new cells.

We must wait approximately two weeks to allow the white blood cells to drop to zero.

Two weeks after the chemotherapy treatment, the two lumps in my neck have diminished significantly! Thank God for that, at least it was worth it!

For the second time, I ask Peter to shave my head! My hair is starting to fall-out again! It is sad and it hurts me so! They were so pretty all curly! Who knows, maybe the next time they grow, they will still curl! And the saga goes on...

VI

The baby blood cells collection...

For the first collection of the new baby blood cells, Peter and I have to be at the hospital for six o'clock in the morning.

They take eight tubes of blood and send them to the laboratory for analysis. They must make sure that the white blood cells are exactly right.

Now we have a two-hour wait; so we go to the cafeteria. After two hours, we return to see if the results are in.

Everything is fine, we can proceed! I go to the Radiology Ward to have the catheter installed. This is a tube they insert in my neck; it has two tubes sticking out (I call them my 'E.T.' ears)! The blood goes out through one of the tubes then passes in a huge machine called: ('Férèse') and runs through eight different pouches that are hanging on that machine. After this 'trip', the blood comes back in my body via the second tube.

The machine sorts the blood cells and only keeps the good baby blood cells that will then be sent to 'HEMA Quebec' to be frozen. This procedure lasts between six to eight hours meaning that I am hooked to this machine for the entire process. The nurse always stays by my side to make sure that all goes well!

In the afternoon, Eric comes for a visit; it helps cut the monotony a bit! Peter and I finally leave the hospital at seven o'clock that night. What a day, we are both so tired! Who would not be after all this...?

This same procedure is repeated five consecutive days. The last day, the Doctor comes to see me and says:
"Unfortunately, we did not collect enough baby blood cells! Your white blood cells are now too high therefore; we cannot get anymore baby blood cells. You will have ten days to rest and recuperate. Hopefully we will have better luck the next time around!"

While he is talking, he retrieves the catheter from my neck because, if left there, it can cause serious infection!

Peter and I are discouraged! To think that we have to go through this again; I cannot stop thinking about the installation of the catheter!

Days like these are very hard on Peter! He sits there waiting day-in day-out... I cannot believe that I will have to go through this again! What else can I possibly do; I did accept the challenge!

After all, we have been through since the beginning of this monstrosity; it is way too late to change my mind now. I said 'yes', so I have to play the game, even if I do not like it! I can honestly say that I am not looking forward to the second round!

The week following the collect of my baby blood cells, the Oncologist schedules an appointment for a liver biopsy. This is a one-day-in-hospital operation! They want to find out if the chemotherapy treatment and the collect of the baby blood cells have affected my liver in any way.

Peter and I go for the pre-op blood tests. Three days later, we arrive at the hospital at six a.m. for the biopsy.

The nurse takes me in a room and asks me to put on the hospital gown. A few minutes later, she returns and installs a serum. After that I am taken down to the Radiology Ward, on a stretcher, for an ultrasound of my stomach, kidneys and spleen. Once the results come back and all the tests are good, the Doctor performs the biopsy.

When they bring me back in the room, the nurse says that I must lie on my right side for two hours. Suddenly, I feel a pain that goes from the incision, into my shoulder and down my arm. I mention this to the nurse and she gives me painkillers. She takes my blood pressure every 15 minutes and finds it very low. She asks me to relax and to try to rest!

Late that afternoon, I am still lying down when the Surgeon comes in. As soon as I see him, I ask:

"When can we go home? We are both so exhausted!"

"We have to wait for your blood pressure to stabilize. Once all is fine, you will be able to go. At home, you must not strain yourself for at least three days to prevent hemorrhage."

A few hours later, finally they allow us to leave. Another trying day for both of us! We spent more than 14 hours at the hospital; Peter and I are completely exhausted!

My guardian Angel calls and says:

"I have scheduled several meetings for you before the beginning of the second collect of your baby blood cells."

She gives me the name of a dietitian saying that she would come by during my second collect adding:

"It is very important that you see a dietitian because there could come a time, during the auto graft, when you will not be able to eat."

We have another meeting with the auto graft specialist and finally we ask our questions to which she answers clearly and we discuss further on the subject. She pursues saying:

"Because of the seriousness of the intervention and also that you will be hospitalized for a long period of time without even being allowed to leave your room, nor open a window, we have two beautiful suites put at your disposition.

81

These private rooms are very well equipped!
They have a huge bathroom that includes a
full-size bathtub. Adjacent to the room, there is
a little living room with comfortable sofas, a
refrigerator, a microwave, a toaster and an
electric kettle for your early coffee. We really
try our utmost best to make your stay as
comfortable as possible and make sure that you
have the necessary equipment to simplify life
during your isolation."

Afterwards, we meet with a psychiatrist
who says that she is available for me at any
time and for Peter and the children should they
find the need. She adds:
"This sickness is not only hard physically; it is
also very hard morally! It is terrifying for your
surrounding to have to deal with this! It is
mostly difficult for your spouse, being with a
sick person 24 hours a day! He may need
comforting and also want to talk with someone
and require support and encouragement."

We meet with the Oncologist eight days
after the first collect of the baby blood cells. He
says:
"Things are looking up! So far, the results
received are all good! The only results that are
missing are the scan and the liver biopsy. They
should not delay much longer! I will call you in
two days and if everything is still good, we will
be able to schedule the second collect of the
baby blood cells. Stay strong, we are on the
right track!"

Two days later and as promised, the Doctor calls and says:
"We can start the second collect of the baby blood cells next Monday. Be at the hospital for eight a.m. for the blood tests. See you then!"

Monday morning, back to the hospital for the second chemotherapy treatment! Then, 'Neupogen' injections for nine days!

The seventh day after the treatment, my guardian Angel calls and says:
"The Radiology Ward will install your catheter ('E.T.' ears) next Tuesday at 7H30 a.m.; simply present yourself at the Ward."

You have no idea how tempted I am to yell 'NO' because I already know how terribly painful it is! Yet, at 7H30 a.m. the following Tuesday, we are back in the hospital!

They start with the blood tests, my poor veins; they are so abused and so tired! Next, to the Radiology Ward for the catheter!

On the way back, we meet the Oncologist who says:
"There will be no collect of your baby blood cells today; the white blood cells are still too low! We will try again tomorrow!"

Home we go with my 'E.T.' ears which, by the way, on top of being extremely painful to install, are also terribly uncomfortable to sleep with!

The next day, my white blood cells are still too low! Therefore, there will be no collect again today!

Finally, the third day, my white blood cells are perfect and they hook me up to the famous machine. Today, for the second round, I have the first collect of baby blood cells!

The fourth day, during the collect of the baby blood cells, the dietitian specialist comes to see me towards the end of the morning. She has a whole bunch of papers in her hands and sits by my bedside. She asks:
"How are your eating habits? Do you eat healthy foods?"

Peter is standing next to me! So I look at him and with a smile, I tell the dietitian:
"Since the beginning of my chemotherapy treatments, the 22nd of January 2002, Peter cooks this special soup that contains a lot of iron and tons of veggies. He blends the whole thing and it becomes a smooth cream; I can easily drink it."

The dietitian gathers her papers and says: "Well, even if you were to have this soup, a few times a day during your stay here, you will be fine. There seems to be sufficient nourishment in this soup to sustain you throughout the entire day."

They repeat the second collect of baby blood cells four days in a row after which they decide that they have enough baby blood cells to proceed with the auto graft.

On the last day of the collect, the Oncologist comes and removes my (E.T.) ears. What a relief!

While he removes the tube, he says:
"We should be able to proceed with the auto graft of the bone marrow in about three weeks. In the meantime, I will make all the necessary arrangements with the auto graft specialist and she will call you back with the details. During these three weeks, I strongly suggest that you rest as much as possible and eat well in order to amass all the strength you can for the difficult period ahead. Tell me, up to now, how do you feel? Are you still willing to pursue with the auto graft?"
"So far, I am a little tired and sometimes, I do find it quite difficult! Nevertheless, I am still very decided to go on with the auto graft!"

Peter and I return home without my E.T. ears! The best news in all this is that we are hospital free tomorrow. Finally, we will be able to sleep-in! What luxury!

We have three full weeks to ourselves. WOW! Awesome! No hospital, no exams and even better, no blood tests. Is this possible? A real vacation!

Peter and I decide to take advantage of these three weeks to the fullest without, of course, forgetting the Doctor's advice.

For Mother's day, Eric invites the whole family for a lobster festival. He opens a magnum of Champagne and we toast to the success of my auto graft! What a magnificent day; simply perfect! I will remember it for the rest of my life!

We also take time to do some shopping because I will be hospitalized for quite a while; therefore, I need a couple of things!

Of course, we go dancing a few times! We honestly do not know how long it will be before we are able to go again!

Rick and Eric take us out to dinner at least once a week and Lily and her family come over as often as they can. All this really helps us get through this rough waiting period!

These three weeks are very precious to us and we do our best to fill every moment of every day up to the roof. We do all we can to try to think less of what lies ahead!

Unfortunately, the three weeks go by way too fast and one morning, the Doctor calls and says:
"All the collected baby blood cells that were frozen are good! The hospital will call you to confirm the date of your admission! From there, we will proceed with the final stage of the auto graft."

VII

The hospitalization...

Exactly two weeks after Mother's day, Peter takes me to the hospital for the auto graft of the bone marrow; it is 3H30 p.m.

WOW! What a room! The auto graft specialist was right when she said that it was huge. It is absolutely terrific! The bathroom with its full size bathtub; everything she mentioned is here!

The nurse comes in and ties the admission bracelet on my wrist! She tells me to take all the time I need to install myself as comfortably as possible.

A few moments later, Eric and his girlfriend arrive and invite us to a Chinese dinner. I love Chinese food! I ask the nurse if I can leave the hospital now that I have been admitted. She replies:
"We have nothing further for you tonight! It would be good if you were back by 8H30 p.m. 'Bon appétit' and enjoy!"

Even though our nerves are on edge, we take full advantage of this outing and enjoy the company. We joke, laugh and try to make the best of our time together! We must appreciate the good things when they come by, notwithstanding what lies ahead!

We return to the hospital a little passed eight p.m. with a doggy bag containing the leftovers of our delicious meal. There is enough for both of us and we will have a very good dinner tomorrow night!

Eric and his girlfriend leave at 8H30 p.m. and while I chat with Peter, I finish placing my things. Peter stays with me; he can feel that I am very nervous! We sit in the comfortable sofas and talk of different things; all except sickness... Around 9H30 p.m. he leaves and I spend the first of my 25 nights in the hospital! This is Sunday, May 25th, 2003.

I had a very restless night and early this morning they take me down, in a wheelchair to install a bigger catheter in my neck. To find words to explain this excruciating pain is impossible! They bring me back on a stretcher and the nurse gives me some painkillers. I sleep most of the day! Thank God I am able to sleep, at least the time that I sleep, I do not feel the pain so much!

Around lunchtime, Eric drops by and finds me asleep! The nurse informs him that she gave me painkillers and that I will be out for at least a few hours. He leaves!

Peter arrives at 4H30 p.m. and we eat our Chinese leftovers which I heated in the microwave. Thank God, the tube is not too close to my throat... Eric comes back after six p.m. and stays until eight o'clock.

The three of us sit in the little living room and chat. This helps me and calms me down! Peter leaves at 9H30 p.m. Of course, being in a private room, my visitors are not limited to regular visiting hours.

After he leaves, the nurse takes blood tests and brings my pills including a sleeping pill; I know that I need one tonight! Tomorrow is a huge day; it is the beginning of the five full days of intensive chemotherapy treatment. Needless to say that I am extremely nervous!

Even with the sleeping pill, I still cannot fall asleep! Finally I doze off at around 2H15 a.m.; but at three o'clock I wake up with a splitting headache! The nurse comes to check on me at five o'clock and I tell her that I have a terrible headache. She takes my blood pressure and gives me an analgesic.

No sooner I doze off; I hear:
"Good morning! It is time for your blood test!"

I am totally awake; it is exactly six a.m.!

I take a nice warm bath after which I am brought down for a lung x ray.

The Hepatitis specialist had prescribed injections before the chemotherapy treatment. The nurse gives me the injections and after, in comes the brigade! We are off and rolling...

The nurse brings the first pouch of chemotherapy and hangs it on the metal rod. For the first day, they take my blood pressure every half-hour! I am very closely surveyed! They want to make sure that all goes well!

The dietitian passes her head through the door and says:

"I hope that you still drink your soup?"

"Yes, of course I do!"

"If you feel like having something from the cafeteria, all you have to do is ask. You are allowed this special treatment!"

"I am honestly not in the mood for anything right now, but thank you very much. I will keep that in mind!"

Early afternoon, Eric arrives and not even an hour later, Lily comes in and they stay with me for a while. It is so wonderful to see them and we talk and talk as though there was no tomorrow. Being isolated does not seem so bad with all these super special visits!

Lily leaves at four and Peter enters half an hour later. In spite of the chemotherapy, I had quite a nice day. To have such great people around me is so fantastic!

It is Wednesday morning and I am still receiving chemotherapy. At 6H30 a.m.:

"Good morning! I am here for your blood test!"

Another day begins! At 9H30 a.m., René-Luc comes in the room and says:

"I came to heat your 'miracle soup' now that you are all hooked-up!"

I drink my hot soup and we chat! I find him very thoughtful to come and see me!

I rediscover the wonderful friendship that we had for so many years when we were young! We could not have chosen a better timing to rekindle the good old days!

At 11H15 a.m., Eric hops in! He explains that he cannot stay very long because he has to attend a luncheon. That is quite all right, at least he comes by and I appreciate it!

I have less appetite now and it goes without saying that I am not hungry at all for lunch! Early in the afternoon, Rick's friend comes by and spends a couple of hours with me. I find that very nice of her to take the time, knowing that she has a very busy schedule. I really appreciate her visit!

After she leaves, the Cardiologist drops by! He examines me and prescribes another electrocardiogram.

I am very tired and yet I still cannot sleep! I am constantly going to the washroom, which of course is very normal with all the liquid that they are pumping into me! After all the commotion of ins and outs, I finally fall asleep and at last, I am able to rest for a little while.

During the treatment, I receive all kinds of medications; some to protect my kidneys, others to prevent the vomiting, some for the Hepatitis and more for my heart. I also receive several injections of immunoglobulin; a protein that stimulates my antibodies.

At 5H30 p.m., Peter arrives! He heats up my soup and we sit in the little living room and chat. Another exhausting day! I hope that to sleep tonight because I really need the rest!

Thursday is the third day of intensive chemotherapy! I slept better last night despite the nine times I had to go to the washroom!

I am getting more and more tired and I tell the nurse about it. She explains:
"You must not worry; this is normal! It is all because of the chemotherapy treatment! As you go along with the auto graft, you will go through different stages. Like I said; do not worry too much, we are keeping a very close eye on you!"

They continue adding different pouches on the metal rod! René-Luc comes earlier this morning! He heats up my soup and stays a little longer. I am already starting to have more difficulty swallowing! It is as though my throat is tightening. The nurse gives me a liquid to dilute in water and I must gargle every hour with this mixture.

Eric comes by at around ten a.m. and spends the rest of the morning with me. Later when my lunch tray arrives, he does his utmost best to encourage me to eat something but it is impossible. I force myself to drink my soup twice a day but even that is becoming more and more difficult!

I find it very hard to get out of bed! I have less strength and I am so tired!

That same afternoon, Lily, Cassandra and Karl-David come for a visit. I try my best to look as good as possible for them but believe me; it is not easy. Overall, it turned out to be quite a nice visit!

Approximately five minutes after they leave, Peter enters and spends the evening with me. Tonight, when the nurse gives me my pills, I cannot swallow them. She grinds them between two spoons and even grinded, it is very difficult to swallow.

My visitors' schedule is perfect! Incredible that only six people (including my 'Mine-Mines') can give me so much support, so much strength and so much love. It is very special and wonderful! Good support is an extraordinary therapy in itself!

Friday, I am on my fourth day of intensive chemotherapy treatment and to say the truth, I do not feel well at all. My appetite is non-existent and when I try to drink my soup, it does not go down. I am incapable of swallowing anything!

I cannot get out of bed! They put a toilet chair beside my bed, because I cannot make it on my own to the washroom. Even though the washroom is only five little steps away from the bed, I cannot make it!

René-Luc arrives as usual around 8H30 a.m. but I feel terrible and I ask him to leave. I even find it hard to talk! I ask the nurse to call Peter for me and, painfully, I tell him:

"Darling, please do not come to the hospital today, I feel so bad! I am more or less drifting in and out of delirium! I am so scared Peter, it is terrible! Please stay home today; it would be best for both of us!"

Eric comes by at lunchtime and I ask him to go! Poor Eric, he leaves the room very worried and the nurses talk with him for a while trying to comfort him.

The nurse comes in and I say:
"I think I have fever!"

No sooner have I said it, I am out again! Around 2H30 p.m., Peter comes in the room and I simply ask:
"Why?"

Slowly he replies:
"Sweetie, pretend that I am not here! Do not exert yourself trying to speak, close your eyes and rest! I simply want you to know that should you need anything, I am sitting right next to you. I am not going anywhere! Do not worry, I am right here!"

He places a chair next to the bed and sits there!

I am in and out of touch and all of a sudden, I remember very clearly saying to myself:
'Girl, prepare yourself, it is probably time to meet your Creator! I honestly do not think that you will see another tomorrow! Your time is up! Keep the courage; the suffering will soon be over for you!'

It is so funny, but I honestly do not remember having been afraid while I was having these thoughts. It simply seemed to be the normal road I had to take! I was not scared at all!

I pass out! I have no recollection of how long I was out, although I remember very clearly thinking to myself as though someone inside was talking to me:
'How can you have such awful and terrible thoughts? What is wrong with you? You only have another 24 to 30 hours left of chemotherapy and then you can rest. You cannot give up now! You have been through so much suffering; you have come so far; think of all who love you and need you! Think of your two precious 'Mine-Mines'!'

As Peter so often says:
"What would they do without their Mamie? The poor Dears, they need you so much!"
'What about Peter? Have you thought about him? How can you abandon him now?'

It is as though the voice came from very far! At that precise moment, I remember reaching out and grabbing Peter's arm, as you reach out for a lifebelt. Out I go again!

When I come to, I notice that it is dark outside! Peter is always sitting by my side and he even tries to give me a little bit of water; unfortunately it comes right out of my mouth! Now it is official; I cannot swallow anything anymore, not even water!

They continue adding new pouches to the metal rod! Up to now, I have seven or eight different kind of medications that are hanging there. During the evening, a Doctor comes to see me and says:

"The nurses have noted in your dossier, that you cannot swallow anything, not even water. If you still cannot eat nor drink your soup tomorrow, we will be forced to nourish you via intravenous. We simply cannot leave you without nourishment!"

He examines my mouth and says:

"Your mouth and throat are swollen and full of ulcers! This is why it is impossible for you to swallow anything!"

Saturday; finally my last day of intensive chemotherapy! I feel a little better this morning although I still cannot swallow anything.

The Doctor returns and says:

"We will start feeding you intravenously today! This liquid will be your food until you can start eating again!"

He hangs a big pouch, containing a thick white liquid, on the metal rod. A few minutes later, René-Luc comes in and wants to heat up my soup. I stop him and say:

"Well my friend, you have lost your job! My mouth and throat are all swollen and covered with ulcers. I cannot swallow a thing! You see that white pouch hanging there, this will be my nourishment for a while; at least until I can start eating again."

96

He sits by the bed and we chat! When he notices that I am becoming tired, he simply decides to leave.

In the afternoon, Eric and his girlfriend come over for a visit. I cannot get out of bed but at least we can talk.

Peter arrives around six p.m. and I ask him to help me to the long chair. I am so fed up of the bed! I cannot sit very long because I get dizzy, but it feels so good to sit up. During the evening, the Doctor comes in and says:
"Well, here is the final pouch of chemotherapy! Are you happy?"
"I would honestly love to celebrate this wonderful moment but it is quite impossible right now! 'Yes' Doctor, I am very happy that it will finally be over!"

Peter leaves a little passed 9H30 that night. At 11H45 p.m., the chemotherapy bag is empty and the nurse comes in to remove it. HURRAH!

What a glorious moment, I did it, I got through it, I am so proud of myself! Even though I am soar all over and still hooked to so many other bags, it still feels fantastic!

Finally, it is finished; the chemotherapy is finished... and I am still alive! What a good and glorious feeling! HALLELUJAH!!! Thank you so much for having been there my Dear God! Without your precious help and the help of my super support team, I would have never made it; of this, I am certain!

Today is Sunday and I slept a little better last night! I feel so liberated simply knowing that the chemotherapy is finished!

As I see René-Luc coming through the door this morning, I tell him:
"It is over! The chemotherapy is finished! Do you realize? I made it! It is finished! No more chemotherapy treatment! I exult, I feel so free, so relieved! I am ecstatic to be here with all of you! Can you understand René-Luc?"
"It is very easy to understand and I am so happy and so very proud of you!"

In the afternoon, Lily and the children come for a visit. It is so good to see them! I have the impression that it has been an eternity since their last visit.

Poor darling, she constantly says that she would like to come more often. I try to make her understand that, with her numerous responsibilities and due to the fact that she lives and works on the South Shore, there is no way she could be at the hospital every day. I am already very happy for the time that she gives me! Even thought I try to reassure her, she still finds it very hard! I understand her but what more can I say.

My sweet little 'Mine-Mines' were allowed to come to see their Mamie today by special permission! Due to the actual situation, they must wear the mask and cannot come close to me; yet it is simply terrific to be able to see them! I am so very happy!

Peter arrives at his usual time; around 5H30 p.m. and tries to make me drink a little bit of water. He would be so happy if I could swallow a little sip! It is simply not possible for the moment; my throat is still not ready!

Eric comes by at nine o'clock this evening. I had not seen him all day. He says:
"Mom, today I took time out to celebrate the end of your chemotherapy! I had a wonderful day! I started my morning with a game of golf and football in the afternoon. Tonight, a couple of friends and I went to a lobster festival. I thought so much of you Mom, knowing how much you love lobster! So my friends and I made a toast to your health with the biggest lobster tails we could find!"
"I am happy to see that, even in these trying moments, you still take time for yourself and have some fun! I know how much you love sports... Darling, one thing we must never forget; life does go on for all of us!"

He is so happy that finally the chemotherapy is finished and that I am able to talk again! I ask them to take me to the long chair for a few minutes; it feels so good to get out of bed!

I have two days of rest before undergoing the graft of my baby blood cells on Tuesday. I need to sleep and build up my strength before the second episode!

VIII

The auto graft of the bone marrow...

Sunday night, while Eric, Peter and I are chatting, an Oncologist comes in saying that he wants to give me an idea of what will occur in the following two days.

He says:

"This will be another trying period for you because all your red and white blood cells, your platelets and also your bone marrow have been destroyed by the intensive chemotherapy treatment. You have been very weakened by it and you are vulnerable to the slightest infection, disease or virus. This is a very dangerous period for you; your immune system is non-existent. From now on, you will have to be very careful! All visitors will have to wear a mask and disinfect their hands before entering the room! No one, but no one with the slightest cough or infection will be allowed in this room! Your grandchildren will not be authorized to visit you during this period.

Because children are often carriers of microbes and viruses; whether from school or from their friends, it would be very risky for you at this time. It is imperative that these rules be respected to the letter! In the actual state of weakness that you find yourself, it is really a matter of life or death for you! Do you understand everything I am saying?"

Thank God that Eric and Peter are with me! We all stare at the Oncologist with wide-open eyes! He scares us with his horde of revelations! We look at one other and are awestruck! The three of us nod to let him know that we understand!

Of course, we all know that I am in an extremely dangerous and very critical period! I say to myself:
'Do I really realize the depth of this entire situation? Maybe I simply do not want to realize how serious all this is! I find this so scary, so agonizing!'

I look at the Oncologist and say:
"Why are you dramatizing so much Doctor? You are frightening us! Is it really necessary?"
"I am saying these things because it is very important and also because they need to be said! You must be made aware of what you are facing! If you do not understand the gravity of your actual situation, how do you expect to take the necessary precautions? Do you know that a simple cold could kill you? Do you realize that you could die? Do you?"

"Doctor, I do understand that you must tell me all these things; that you must expose me to all the risks I am facing. It is your duty to inform me and I thank you! However, right now, I do not want to hear nor think about all that can happen! First, because if I start thinking of this or that, if I start thinking that I might or might not die, what will be left for me to hang on to? What hope will I have left? Can you understand that, Doctor? Can you try to put yourself in my place? Can you try to understand my point of view? Can you understand that I am scared stiff? Please, I really do not need to hear all this! I absolutely cannot and will not let myself go to these thoughts! I cannot afford it; not now! I need all the strength I can hold on to!"

He raises his arms in despair! At least that is the way I perceived his gesture! More gently, he says:
"Tuesday morning I will be giving you, via transfusion, the first half of your baby blood cells that have already been frozen. I use the syringe method; I prefer it to the other methods! You must not worry about anything; all will go very well! By the way, tomorrow I would like to come with nine students! The auto graft of the bone marrow is part of their training course and I would like them to live the experience. Do you mind?"
"Of course not, Doctor! After all, they are our future doctors and if it helps, why not!"

"Wednesday another Doctor will be giving you the second half of your baby blood cells. He will choose his own method! I think that all is said, all is well, and therefore I bid you all goodnight! All you have to do is rest, I shall see you tomorrow!"

After this, he simply turns around and leaves! The three of us are awe and we stare at the door that is closing behind him! Needless to say that our minds are actually working overtime...

I cannot let myself be demoralized with all this! Otherwise, I will never pull through this! I am conscious that all is far from over, but I absolutely must keep positive thoughts. We all must keep our strength and our energy if we want to at least, have a chance to succeed! I have to continue hoping and praying, as I have been doing all along!

It is incredible, I am shaking and I am so upset! The three of us cannot stop talking about what the Doctor told us. Eric and Peter try to calm me down as much as they can! It is almost 11 p.m. when they decide to leave! They are both so worried, so desperate!

Needless to say that I did not sleep a wink last night! I guess I was still too nervous and had too much going on in my mind!

Monday morning, I ask the nurse to help me because I want to take a long hot bath. It feels so good and it relaxes me! No sooner am I out of the tub, René-Luc comes in.

As soon as he sees me, he notices that I am very preoccupied and decides to stay and chat a little longer. I must keep myself busy today; I do not want to have too much time to think! I am so scared; I feel as though I am in a noose and it is tightening more and more!

I tell him about last night and everything the Doctor told us. He knows the critical phase I am in right now and he is very much aware of the danger I am facing. After listening to me, he says:
"You know, you are a very strong person and also very stubborn! (He says the last word with a smile; after all he does know me from way back!) Try not to think about it too much! Everything will go well! You will pull through this; I know it! You must continue your fight and keep the courage. I know that this is easy for me to say, but you are not alone, we are right here with you! You must stay strong!"

I know that they are all with me and this gives me the strength and courage to fight even more. The fright tortures me so! After René-Luc leaves, I try to make a little siesta! As I start dosing off, in comes the Oncologist with his nine training students! He explains the entire process of the auto graft of the bone marrow and gives them the detail of each pouch that is on the metal rod. He invites them to come back tomorrow morning to assist to the transfusion of the first 12 frozen bags of my baby blood cells.

After talking a mile a minute, the Oncologist turns towards me and very seriously says:
"You should not worry, everything will be fine! Try to rest."

The nine students look at me and smile! The Doctor turns and leaves the room followed by his suite. Before passing the door, the students give me the thumbs-up and together they say:
"Good luck, Madame!"

I thought it was very kind of them and it made me feel better!

In the afternoon, I try to rest, but it is totally impossible! I simply cannot relax! I am way too nervous and even if I do my best to control it, I cannot stop wondering about what is waiting for me tomorrow!

Peter arrives around five p.m.! I am still lying in bed and he sits next to me! Inevitably, we talk about all that is going on! Realizing that this does not help me at all, we decide that it would best to change the subject. Laughingly, I look at Peter and say:
"Darling, why not talk about romance?"

We both burst out laughing! It feels good to laugh even for no reason whatsoever!

In the course of the evening, the nurses come in for several blood tests and they take my blood pressure every half-hour. They bring me down for a lung x ray. It feels good to be amongst people again...

I am still not finished! The cardiology technician comes in the room and passes me an electrocardiogram. I do hope that this will be all; I have really had my share of injections and exams for today!

The nurse returns and injects me a tranquillizer! While doing so, she says: "This should help calm you down for tomorrow! I will be back later with your sleeping injection!"

After all the back-and-forth, the room is finally quiet! Peter and I continue talking for a little while and he leaves!

Tuesday, June 3, the first D-day! In spite of everything the nurse injected me last night to help calm me down, sleep was scarce and I am still very tense! At 7H22 a.m., my blood tests are done, I took a nice hot bath, my bed is made and 'URI' (the name the head-nurse gave my white teddy bear) is sitting on the pillows and overlooking the situation!

The room fills up: the four nurses that take care of me every day; the Oncologist's assistant; then a woman comes in with a box, on wheels, (the size and shape of a small refrigerator) containing my twelve frozen pouches of baby blood cells and three of the nine students that were chosen to assist. Five minutes later, the Oncologist arrives.

He is a happy-go-lucky-person; he always smiles and makes jokes! In a situation like this, believe me it helps a great deal!

106

We are now on a roll and it is a go! The Oncologist takes a syringe while the woman takes out a frozen bag of my baby blood cells and shakes it gently. Once the blood starts to liquefy, the Oncologist fills up the syringe, inserts the needle in the catheter and empties the syringe very fast. I have now received the first bag of my own baby blood cells!

What a bizarre feeling! First; it is very cold as it goes through the tube into my vein and second; I get a very strange taste in my mouth and my mouth becomes watery. To say the truth, I do not feel so hot! I feel like throwing up! God, help me! There are still eleven bags left, notwithstanding the twelve bags of tomorrow! Dear Lord, will I make it through this ordeal?

This procedure goes on throughout the morning! I am totally bushed! When you feel as bad as I do right now, believe me, half a day is like an eternity!

Finally, they all leave the room! The nurse injects me a medication saying:
"This will help you relax and should also make you feel better!"

Not even half an hour later, Eric arrives! I can see in his eyes that he is very worried! He asks how it went this morning and how I feel! He also asks if he can do anything at all for me! Poor Darling, he is so nervous! He stays with me a few minutes but soon realizes that I am very tired and he leaves.

A few minutes after Eric has left me, in comes the nurse and she asks me how I am feeling! To say the truth, I do not feel well at all! She checks my pulse, takes my blood pressure and adds:
"I will talk to the Oncologist and ask him if he could prescribe a stronger tranquillizer for tomorrow's transfusion."

I cannot get out of bed! I even need help to get to the toilet-chair that is next to the bed! I feel terrible and so weak!

Around four o'clock, Lily arrives! She too is very worried! I try to get up to sit with her, no way, my head is spinning! She sits next to the bed and tries to talk with me! Because of the medication, the nurse injected me a little earlier, I tend to doze off. After a few minutes, she leaves! She is terribly sad and would so much like to be able to do more!

Shortly after, Peter comes in and he too is very concerned! We are all trying to hang in there as strongly as we can and we try to give one another as much strength and courage as possible. Whether we want to admit it or not, I am actually crossing a very critical period in my life and I honestly do not know if I am going to pull through this!

At times, especially at night when I cannot sleep, I ask myself; is it all worth it; the pain, the suffering, the worry and the anxiety this causes everyone? I really wonder; is it all worth it! Then, I say to myself:

'My Good Lord, you have made me come this far, you have helped me endure all this pain! Please do not abandon me now! I promised I was going to fight this deadly sickness with all my might and by gosh, I will fight it to the end! I admit that I am very scared and I really need your precious help! I simply cannot make it without You!'

I think it is very normal to have doubts, moments of discouragement, to be scared stiff and to want the whole thing to stop, once and for all... I do not know what I would give for all this to simply go away!

When we stop to think about it, life is such a glorious gift, such a precious gift! How can I even think of not fighting to the utmost in order to keep it? I so much want to take full advantage of this beautiful and wonderful life! Most of all, I want to be with my loved ones more than anything in the whole world! Again, I say to myself:

'The day I was diagnosed, in December 2001, I took the decision to fight with all my might against this deadly sickness. Well girl, now is the time to see what you are made of! You must fight as hard as you can, and fight I will! I must succeed, I simply must!'

Second D-day: Wednesday, 7H09 a.m. My heart is pounding very fast! I keep wondering how the second portion of my transfusion will go today! Another Oncologist will perform it.

When he comes into the room, he explains the method he will use:

"I do not use syringes! I attach the bag of your baby blood cells directly to the tube in your neck. In my point of view, this method is better and a lot faster! Of course, every Doctor has their way of proceeding and in reality; each method is as good as the other!"

When I receive the first bag of my blood cells, I feel this huge pain in my throat; my saliva turns in my mouth! My God, I am going to throw up! It is horrible; I do not feel well at all! My throat is very soar; I cannot stand this pain! My God, I am going to faint! This method is one thousand times worse than yesterday's! I cry out:

"Stop, please stop! I am going to throw up!"

The nurse rushes and puts a tray next to my mouth! The Doctor looks at me and sees that I am not doing well at all. He stops everything and asks the nurse to give me a tranquillizer to help me. Unfortunately, the tranquillizer has no effect whatsoever! Thank God, I did not throw up!

The Doctor continues the transfusion, but this time, he takes his time. He constantly looks at me and asks if I am all right!

Finally, the ordeal is finished! I have the impression that the twelve bags of my blood cells are stuck in my throat!

I am so grateful and happy to see everyone leave the room!

Two hours after they all leave the room, the fever starts!

The nurse had already informed me that I would have fever, but I never imagined it would be so soon.

They immediately start taking blood tests several times a day to make cultures of the blood. Depending on the results of the cultures, they most probably will discover what kind of infection causes me all this fever. It would also help them to give me the right medication to counter it.

I am sure that the fact that my mouth and throat are totally infected with ulcers and are very soar, that surely must be one reason for the infection. I cannot swallow anything! As the day goes on, the fever rises and I feel worse and worse!

Towards the end of the morning, Eric comes to see me, but he does not stay very long; I am totally knocked out! Lily calls every day, sometimes even two and three times a day to ask how I feel!

The phone rings; it is René-Luc with a hoarse voice. He says:
"I have a soar throat and I went to see my Doctor! This morning I passed by the hospital and the nurse refused to let me enter your room. She said that this is really not the time for you to be in contact with someone sick. She also told me not to come back before I am completely cured. Not before!"

"Now I understand why I have not seen you in such a long time! Actually, the nurse is right you know, I have high fever and they do not know what causes it. Right now, my antibodies are non-existent because of the intensive chemotherapy I received. I absolutely have nothing left to fight back even the slightest virus. It is a dangerous period for me, I am already so infected!"

"I understand; the nurse gave me a thorough explanation this morning! I will call you back tomorrow to see how you feel. Keep the courage and take good care of yourself!"

Around five p.m., Peter comes in and finds me still lying in bed. I tell him that my fever is very high and that I feel very drowsy. He sits next to me! To say the truth, I am more out of touch than in...

Today was a very bad day for me and I think to myself:

'Dear God, if at all possible, I beg you to give me a better tomorrow!'

Thursday, the fever still goes higher even with all the antibiotics they inject me.

The nurse comes in and says:

"When the Doctor opened the meeting this morning, he said:

'Now let us talk about the 'burning patient' in room 6'...'"

I want to laugh, but I cannot. He has a right to say that; my fever reached 40.8° this morning. That is hot!

At lunchtime, Eric comes for a visit! I feel too bad to even keep him company. Sad and worried, he leaves!

Towards the end of the afternoon, Peter comes in the room. He finds me very pale and weak! I tell him that I have no energy whatsoever! He sits next to me and tries to distract me by talking about the day he had. No luck, nothing seems to help!

The nurse regularly takes blood tests, my blood pressure and my temperature and hopes for a change. No change whatsoever!

There is always someone in the room; a nurse, a doctor, a technician, always someone! Needless to say that this makes me even more aware of the seriousness of my case!

The wheel of horror begins to turn; the apprehension, the doubts, the fright, the anguish, thus bringing an abundance of questions to my head. I start thinking:
'Am I going to make it? I fought so hard, I have been through so much, I have come so far and yet, I cannot help but ask myself: Will I pull through this? Will I ever get well again? Will this sickness ever leave me?'

It is as though Peter can read my mind! He does not want to leave tonight! He knows that I am in a dangerous impasse right now and he is very scared. He is worried and sad and feels helpless that he cannot make it better. He does not want to leave, but it is already passed ten p.m. and he has to go!

The nurse comes in with my injections for the night. Peter kisses me and leaves! After giving me the injections, she takes more blood tests, my blood pressure and my temperature. Finally, the nurse leaves the room.

I am so sad to see Peter like this! I know and feel all their suffering! Even if they do their utmost best not to show me how much they hurt, I feel it inside me.

I try to sleep, but sleep will not come! I lie there in an incoherent state and the cinema keeps rolling in my head.

Unfortunately, the Good Lord did not seem to hear my prayer last night! Today has not been good at all! Actually, I think that, so far, today has been the worst day of my entire life! Even if things are very bad right now, I know that You are still watching over me and I thank You with all my heart. Once again, Dear Lord, I do pray that you will give me a better tomorrow!

Friday, my fever is still over 40°! I cannot talk anymore, I cannot keep my eyes open and I cannot even sleep! I am so full of medication, I feel so drugged and I cannot think straight. Even with everything they inject me, sleep still does not come! I have the impression that if I fall asleep, I might not wake up! I am in a delirious state and my body and my mind do not want to function anymore!

Eric comes by and sees the Doctor in the corridor. He asks him:

"Tell me Doctor, how is my Mother?"
"Your Mother is very ill! She is actually in a highly critical phase! It could go one way or the other, it is impossible to predict. We are doing our utmost best to save her life! If you have faith Sir, the best thing to do is to pray for her! I cannot tell you more; we are all waiting, hoping and praying for the best."

A few minutes later, Lily arrives and she sees the Doctor. She asks him the same question and the Doctor gives her the same answer. He adds:
"Your brother is in the room with her now."

With great efforts to contain herself, because she wants to try to help her 'little' brother, she enters the room. When she sees me lying there, so pale and motionless, she looks at Eric and bursts out into tears.

Eric takes her in his arms and calms her! They both go out of the room because they do not want me to hear them cry. The Doctor and the nurses talk to them and try to calm them.

After a while, they both come back in the room! They sit next to the bed and hold my hand. I have no reaction whatsoever and they decide to leave. They are sad, worried and very scared that the worse might happen...

Early that afternoon, Peter arrives and sits next to me. I am a little aware of his presence and I try to tell him to go home. I feel so terrible and it is extremely painful for me to even try to talk.

Very calmly, Peter says:
"Cookie, try not to talk, you will hurt yourself for no reason. Close your eyes and rest! I am right here next to you and I am not going anywhere. Remember Sweetheart, you are not alone!"

He places a chair next to the bed and tries to look at the television, but he cannot even concentrate; he is too preoccupied and worried about me!

I have no idea of how long he stayed there, but a few times I felt he was holding my hand. I guess he was trying to give me enough strength and energy to keep me going from hour to hour...

The delirium takes over and the questions start all over again:
'Will I survive this? Will I see another tomorrow? God, I feel so bad...'

At times, I have the impression that I am dying! In my lucid moments, I cannot stop myself from thinking that this is what dying must feel like!

What a bizarre feeling! I am lying there lifeless; one moment I am breathing and the next, I am dying!

Even if I try to fight this unpleasant sensation with all my might and all my willpower, I simply cannot! My brain does not function anymore and my limbs will not obey me at all. It is as though the fever has taken hold of my entire body!

To be honest, I remember very little of this awful period of my sickness! I only have a few glimpses of those horrible eight days. I was more unconscious than awake! I hardly remember the visits I received during that time! I remember very scarcely when Peter came in and kept repeating:
"Cookie, close your eyes and try to rest!"

Everything seems to be so far in my memory! This period is like a blur, like a very thick cloud!

I do not remember having been aware that the Doctor had talked with the children, nor do I remember having heard them cry. To say the truth; I think that it was a lot better this way! I would have suffered too much had I been fully conscious!

I remain several days in this lethargic state! The fever stays at its climax of 40.8° during several days. It remains at over 40° for more than one week.

During this lapse of time, I am always fed intravenously. Several times a day, they take blood tests for cultures. My poor veins, they are so soar and so tired!

In one of the blood analyses, they discover that I have diabetes. I have never had diabetes in my entire life! Yet, the monitor shows 21.4! If you know anything about diabetes; 21.4 is quite high!

The Doctor sees Lily, Eric and Peter and he explains the meaning of this:

"Diabetes is characterized by the presence of excessive amounts of sugar in the urine and manifested by various metabolic disorders of the system. The liquid that she is fed with causes this; it is very concentrated! We will start giving her insulin injections four times a day. We absolutely need to follow this very closely and do everything we can to control it!"

Lily and Eric ask the Doctor:
"Can you not feed her anything else to bypass the diabetes?"
"Unfortunately, we do not have a huge variety of menus for intravenous meals! This does happen sometimes! As I was saying, what we feed her is very concentrated. I am sure that this is temporary and it will resolve to normal once she starts eating on her own. Of course, we must follow this closely because it could become dangerous. We have started insulin injections four times a day and we take blood tests on a regular basis. For the time being, we must continue feeding her in his manner; we do not have any other choice."

Eric looks at the Doctor and asks him:
"Doctor, do you have any idea if or when things will ever become normal?"

Poor Doctor, what can he say, he cannot even lie, he honestly does not know what is going to happen himself. The doctors and the nurses are really doing their utmost best to try to save my life. What more can he say? He raises his arms, turns around and leaves...

For more than a week, I do not know whether it is day or night! I am in a delirium phase and the fever stays high. I feel as though I am in a tunnel and there is no way out; only darkness!

Peter and the children come to the hospital every day! They constantly fear that something will occur! It is very hard on all of them; they feel so helpless... They try to see the Doctor as often as possible and question him.

Because there is no change in the temperature, the diabetes or my general condition, he does not have much to say. Like all of them, he continues to wait and hope...

After a full week of not knowing what is happening around me; the following Saturday, I become a little more awake.

I have more moments that are lucid; I even start talking a little! I can keep my eyes open a little longer; but I am still too weak to get up!

They still feed me intravenously and I am still diabetic! Fortunately, my diabetes is going down a little because of the insulin injections they give me four times a day.

Saturday night, Peter comes as usual and admires my effort to smile! Although I still must keep the bed, he in turn has a big smile on his face and is very happy to see me a little more alive. He says that my eyes are brighter and that I even have a few colors. He sits near the bed and takes my hand!

There is still hope for me! I am slowly coming back to life and I can honestly tell you that it is divine!

Peter always has this obsession to see me overcome this sickness! He constantly thinks about it and holds on to this thought as a drowning person would hold on to a lifebelt. The smallest smile, the slightest word I pronounce, everything and anything I do gives him hope and encourages him...

Sunday morning, I feel a little better than yesterday! René-Luc, who is now totally cold and fever free, enters the room wearing a mask. At first, I do not recognize him! I look more closely and laughingly I say:

"I did not recognize you! It must be because I have not seen you in such a long time and with the disguise..."

"My Doctor assured me that I was totally cured! The nurse allowed me to come in on the conditions that I wear the mask and that I do not come close to you."

"I find it a little easier to talk today and I do not feel as groggy! The nurse told me, earlier this morning that my fever had started to drop a little bit. You know, I went way up to 40.8°! In one of the meetings, the Oncologist even described me as the 'burning patient'; can you imagine? This morning when the nurse took my temperature, miraculously, it was down to 39.7°. Believe me; compared to 40.8°, what a huge improvement..."

We talk for a while and as soon as he sees that I am getting tired; he decides to leave and let me rest!

A little before lunch, Eric and his girlfriend come for a visit. I ask Eric to help me to the long chair even if only for a few minutes. I really need to get out of that bed. I must say that the change is heavenly!

Ten minutes later, I have to go back to bed! My head is starting to spin and I am tired. We continue talking a little but very soon, they have to leave.

No sooner have they gone, I doze off! I guess it was good to get out of bed!

The nurse wakes me up for my diabetes check and I realize that I slept nearly two hours. It really did me a lot of good!

Later that afternoon, as soon as Peter arrives, I ask him to help me to the long chair. This time I stay a little longer! He sits next to me and we chat while I rest from the bed.

Slowly, I seem to be coming back to life and what an extraordinary good feeling! Thank You Dear Lord, from the bottom of my heart, for everything You do for me! I will never thank You enough for having given me such a wonderful group of people to surround me in these terrifying moments. They are all so incredible and without You and my super team, I would have never made it this far! In fact, I am sure that I would no longer be part of this beautiful world!

Monday, I have several blood tests; one for the Hepatitis, one for the diabetes and another one in preparation for a scan that the Doctor had prescribed. My poor veins are suffering! With all the chemotherapy I had, my veins have hardened and it has become very difficult for the technicians to get the amount of blood they need every morning.

René-Luc comes for a visit in the morning to heat up my 'miracle soup' and Eric comes every day around lunchtime.

This afternoon, Lily and the 'Mine-Mines' come to see me; it has been quite a while since the last visit of my little Darlings. The Doctors had mentioned that, because of the high fever, they would not be allowed to come to the hospital. What great therapy they are for me! Although they cannot come close and that I cannot even hug them; simply seeing them lifts my spirits! They give me so much strength, energy, courage and love!

They keep staring at me and when Lily notices it, she explains that they have been so worried and to see me sitting and smiling, simply makes them very happy.

Again tonight, as every other night since I have been hospitalized, Peter arrives. He looks at me with his tender smile and is very happy to see that I am feeling better, that I am more awake and that I look better. Compared to last Friday, he simply cannot get over the huge progress I have made!

He is overwhelmed and cannot help but show his immense joy! Peter offers me some water and even though it is still very painful, I succeed in swallowing a few drops. Another wonderful victory to my credit!

Try to imagine; after having gone through such an ordeal, after fighting so hard, after hanging on night after night, after being so scared of dying, for Peter to see me like this is such a great relief, such a good feeling for him! He cannot begin to express how happy he is and how proud he is of me. He simply looks at me and smiles!

Peter and Eric have not missed one day since I have been hospitalized! They were always here thru thick and thin!

Lily was not able to come to the hospital every day, but she came as often as she possibly could. She called every day, sometimes even three times a day. That is so awesome! We must not forget that she has a full-time job, two children and numerous responsibilities notwithstanding that she is the only one that lives on the South Shore. René-Luc who also works full-time and even through his cold and fever period, called every day and always found time to be there for me.

When I stop to think about it, I cannot get over the fact that only four people can give me so much strength, so such courage, so such encouragement and so much love, I find this incredible!

Do not worry, I am certainly not forgetting my sweet little 'Mines-Mines' who are the sun and joy of my life! I must admit that despite their young age, like us they really do their best to get through these trying times. They are both extraordinary!

Rick is a precious asset to his Father! He calls him nearly every day and constantly encourages him. Although he travels a lot, he tries his best to see him as often as possible. What a great support for Peter! Lord knows that Peter, who constantly gives, also needs support and understanding. It is fine to give but one must receive once in a while...

Tuesday, June 18th, this is my 24th day in the same 'cloistered' room! Even if it is a very nice suite and fully equipped; nevertheless, it remains a hospital room and I am in total isolation.

Other than the nurses, the doctors, the technicians, my visitors and the four walls that surround me; I have absolutely no contact with the outside world. I am not even aloud to open a window, let it be to breathe a little bit of outside air...

Of course, you might say:
'Well, there is always the television!'

To tell you the truth, nothing on television seems to interest me! With all the activity that I have day in, day out, I prefer to keep my strength for more important things, especially for my precious visitors.

This morning the nurse comes in, hands me a glass of lukewarm liquid and asks me to try to drink it. As I did last night, I drink it very slowly! She takes my temperature and with a nice smile on her face, she shouts out gladly:

"Miraculously, it is down to 37.8°! Do you believe this? We have not seen this in such a long time! I am so happy for you!"

After which she adds:

"I will ask the Doctor if we can start giving you some chicken broth a few times a day. This would be the ideal way to start eating again thus getting rid of your intravenous feeder and reducing your diabetes."

As soon as she leaves and without losing one second, I jump on the phone and call Peter. I tell him that the nurse is going to ask the Doctor if they can start giving me some chicken soup. Needless to say it did not take more for him to reply:

"I am so happy and proud of you! I will come over shortly and bring a nice thermos of hot chicken soup, my recipe. Does this remind you of something?"

"Oh yes, I remember that famous night when you crossed the entire city, in a big snow storm, to bring me a thermos of hot chicken soup when I had my bad laryngitis and I hardly had any voice left. Is this the event you are referring to Darling?"

"Yes, that is exactly it!"

René-Luc comes in, no mask this time and finds me sitting in the long chair! He can hardly believe his eyes and says:

"When I think that only last Friday you were in such critical condition and to see you like this today, what a miracle! You have started to drink a little; you are sitting in your chair with a nice smile that passes from one ear to the other. You have no idea how happy I am for you! We were all so afraid of losing you!"

The conversation is very nice and we even allow ourselves a few jokes. It feels so good to laugh a little and to feel in better shape. It has been such a long journey!

After his visit, a parade of doctors comes in; two Oncology specialists, the Hepatitis specialist, the Cardiologist and believe it or not, even a Psychiatrist.

It is as though they had established a schedule: one leaves and another one comes in. All these 'nice' visits take place in one single morning!

They are all very puzzled by the behavior of my cancer! I seem to be a real mystery to every one of them! They ask so many questions and require so many tests to an extent that I ask myself:

'Am I still in a critical stage?'

Finally, the room is quiet! The nurse comes in with a tray; I have not seen one of those in quite a while! It is a cup of lukewarm chicken broth! She says:

"Drink it very slowly and try to drink as much as you can. This is very good for you! "

Thanks to this 'famous' chicken broth, I slowly start eating again. It feels wonderful and I add one more great victory to the list!

IX

The transfer...

Early afternoon, the Oncologist enters the room with a smile on his face and says:
"I have been in a meeting all morning with the Oncology specialist team and after discussing your case thoroughly, we came to the conclusion that it would be time to transfer you to a semi-private room. Your fever is very close to normal. Last night, the nurse brought you some lukewarm chicken broth and you were able to swallow a few sips thus meaning that the infections in your mouth and in your throat are clearing up quite well. Your blood cells are coming along very well; therefore, your antibodies will become stronger and stronger. Your diabetes level has already started to come down and the sooner you start eating, the sooner we will be able to stop feeding you intravenously thus finally bringing your sugar level back to normal. We can very well keep you under observation in a semi-private room!

128

We have to liberate this room for another patient who is waiting for his graft. We will transfer you during the evening, thus giving you time to prepare yourself. You must take all the time you need; you are still very weak you know! What do you have to say about my proposition? Does it please you?"

"Doctor, this is the best news I have heard in a very long time and I thank you from the bottom of my heart. I am nearly tempted to give you a big hug to show you all my gratitude; but please do not worry Doctor, I will control myself!"

He looks at me and we both burst out laughing!

I can hardly contain myself! I am so anxious to get on the phone and give this great news to all my loved ones. I know how pleased and happy they will be and Lord knows that they need to hear good news after having been through so much...

Thank God, shortly after the Doctor leaves, Eric comes in. I must say that I am relieved to see that this is not another Doctor! I have nothing against the Doctors, they are all wonderful, but honestly; I have had my share of Doctors!

The way Eric looks at me; I can see the relief on his face and the happiness in his eyes. It is as though he already knows that something special and good has happened! Today, I really feel that I am a gift for him!

For the first time, in such a very long time, I do not see fear nor sadness in his eyes! This time, I can see joy and tenderness! If only you knew how relieved and happy this makes me; you cannot imagine!

I feel like a million bucks! All excited and with a big smile, I tell Eric everything the Doctor mentioned during his visit! I talk about the transfer in a semi-private room that will take place tonight and also that I will finally be taken out of my 'cloister' room and back amongst people.

He listens very closely! Without even having asked him anything, he starts gathering all my things so that I will be ready when they come to transfer me tonight. He waits until I finish drinking all my chicken broth before leaving. I ask him to help me back into bed; I am tired! It is very comprehensible after all this excitement and this great joy! This time when he leaves, he is happy and in peace!

I must have slept at least a few hours because when Peter arrives, around 5H30 holding our biggest thermos in his hands, he wakes me up. Needless to say that I knew what was in the thermos!

Peter sees the luggage by the door and asks me what is going on! I tell him about the Doctor's visit and the transfer to a semi-private room. I ask him to help me to the chair and to give me a cup of hot broth. He is very happy not have to force me to drink it!

While I slowly sip my hot chicken soup, I give Peter all the details of the super busy day I had. He is sitting by my side and listens to every word! His face is all smiles and his eyes are sparkling! When I finally stop talking, he says:

"Sweetie, this is one of the most beautiful days in my entire life! To see you like this, smiling and recounting your day all excited, to have you sitting here close to me for longer than only a few minutes, to see you so lively and happy; I cannot begin to tell you how very proud I am of you! You fought so hard, went through so much pain, so much anguish and so much fear, this is incredible. When I think of the critical stage you were in only last Friday, and to see you like this today, it warms my heart. It is a real miracle! I can hardly believe it; it simply seems too good to be true! I am so happy and so proud of you!"

We cannot stop talking! Time goes by so fast and suddenly we realize that it is passed ten p.m. and no one has come to transfer me. Peter would like to help me get installed in the new room but it is so late; he has no choice but to leave. Finally, he kisses me and goes!

A few minutes after Peter's departure, two nurses enter the room; one is pushing a wheelchair and asks me to sit in it while the other nurse picks up the luggage and off we go! I am out in the open and driven to my semi-private room!

131

After being cloistered for so long in an isolation room, I find myself back in the 'circulation' amongst people and even better; I do not have to wear a mask. What an extraordinary sensation! Even more so, what a glorious victory!

Even if I tried very hard to express my emotions or to explain what I am feeling right this minute, while rolling towards my semi-private room, I honestly could not find the words. I cannot stop looking everywhere, I smile at all the people I see on the way; it is incredible! It feels as though I have recovered my freedom! God this is so good!

Needless to say that I did not sleep much that night! Firstly, because I am too excited and I cannot stop my mind from rewinding everything that has happened to me today and secondly, because I find this new room a lot noisier than the other one! Most of all, it is because I cannot stop thinking that now that I am out of isolation and in a semi-private room, soon, very soon, I will be able to go home. This is the thought that totally occupies my mind. For all these reasons, I cannot keep my eyes closed; therefore, I cannot fall asleep!

I am so anxious to go back to our little nest, to sleep in my own comfortable bed, to go wherever I please, whenever I please. The simple fact of going home will probably be the biggest, the greatest victory of all since the beginning of this terrifying sickness.

My joy seems contagious! Every person I meet on the way looks at me and gives me a huge smile!

Wednesday morning, six o'clock, in comes the technician with her basket full of syringes, tampons, etc. and she says:

"Good morning! It is time for your blood test!"

I greet her with a nice big smile! She seems surprised to see me smile this way. She says:

"I have to admit dear Madame, that I am rarely received with such a beautiful smile, especially at six o'clock in the morning!"

We both burst out laughing! As soon as she finishes taking my blood test, she goes towards the other bed and in comes the diabetes technician. She pokes me and checks the monitor. Totally surprised, she looks at me and says:

"This is very good! The monitor indicates that you are now testing at 9.7. When we compare to the 21.4 that you tested the first time, you have made enormous progress. This is really very impressive!"

After they both leave, in comes another nurse and she too has a nice smile! She places a chair in the washroom and comes towards me saying:

"This morning, you will try to wash yourself alone. If you cannot make it alone, I will come and help you. Take all the time you need! For the first time, you should not rush!"

Needless to say that I will do my utmost best to succeed on my own! I might sound funny to you to even mention this; after all, to wash ourselves is a very normal thing!

Ever since that famous Friday after the auto graft of the bone marrow, it has mostly been the nurses who have washed me in bed every morning. I am certain that now you understand why I really want to succeed in this task. It will allow me to add another victory to my now longer list of victories!

I have to admit that it took me quite a long time to complete my task but I did it all alone, like a 'big girl'. I was totally bushed but very proud of myself! No one rushed me; to the contrary, as the nurse had said, they gave me all the time I needed.

Shortly after, the four wonderful nurses, that took such good care of me during my long stay in isolation, come to see me one after the other. They congratulate me for having passed through this ordeal, they wish me the best of luck and they sincerely hope to never see me in their ward again...

They all found me very patient! They wish they would have more patients like me in the future. I am very happy not to have caused them too much trouble even in the worse periods of the graft.

I express my extreme gratitude for all that they have done for me and for their constant patience and I add:

"To every one of you, please accept my most sincere 'THANK YOU' from the bottom of my heart for all the time and the attention you have given me. Without only one of you, I would have never made it through this awful sickness! Again many many thanks!"

We all have tears in our eyes! We hug and they return to fulfill their precious duties. I thought it was so kind and nice of them to take the time to come and see me like this. It really warmed my heart!

What a wonderful team they make! They really have the vocation of their trade! Lord knows that it is not easy to do what they do and this, day after day! They surely have extraordinary nerves and they must all be extremely strong!

After all these wonderful visits, breakfast is served; a bowl of porridge, hot milk and toasts. I was unable to eat the toast, but I did eat a little bit of porridge. My God, it feels so good to eat!

Today, everything I do is nice, everything is good and everything is positive! I am at the peak of happiness! I am euphoric!

René-Luc enters the room and with a smile says:
"I went to the other room and all the nurses were very happy to inform me that you had been transferred last night. What good news, I am so happy for you! Now that you are part of the 'society' when will you be going home?"

"I have not yet received my release! The Doctor told me he wanted to keep me under observation a little longer to see how things will go. I imagine it should not be too long before he sends me home! If only you knew how happy I am to be back in the 'society' as you say! I see all these smiling faces and I am so proud to be the cause of all this happiness! If only you knew how good it feels to look at smiling faces instead of constantly seeing sadness and fear in everyone's eyes; you have no idea! After all the worrying and the suffering we have all been through; these smiling faces are a huge reward for me! I feel like an Olympic champion who has won her first gold medal! What an accomplishment! What a formidable sensation! Can you understand my excitement and the immense joy I am living right now?"

"I understand you very well and you have all the reasons in the world to be proud after all you have been through. If there is one person on this earth who deserves to be happy and proud, that person is you! If only you knew how happy and proud I am of you!"

Because my 'new' room is very small and compact compared to the suite I had before, René-Luc has no choice but to leave when my Doctor makes his entrance with a huge smile on his face. The Doctor acknowledges René-Luc, turns towards me and as usual, goes right to the point saying:

"Your blood tests are good, your diabetes has come down drastically and you have no more fever. Also, very important, you have even started to eat a little revealing that the infection in your mouth and throat are getting better. If this keeps up during the day, we think that you should be able to go home tomorrow. What do you think of that?"

"Oh Doctor, this sounds like beautiful music to my ears! You have no idea how anxious I am to go back home, it has been so long! I promise that I will be very good!"

"Of course, you will be in convalescence for at least six months. You will have to take very good care of yourself. You must rest a lot, have good and healthy meals, and eat regularly. Even if you do not eat much at the beginning, at least eat something and eat more often during the day. You will get tired very fast. You certainly will not be able to do much once you get home but do not force it, you must take the time to rebuild your strength. After all that, you have been through; you must understand that all these precautions are absolutely necessary. Your system has been abused and totally destroyed by all the chemotherapy you have received and you will need to be very careful! You are still very weak and fragile and you will be in this state for quite a while. Force yourself to eat more and more every day and do not forget to rest as much as you can. All this is imperative to recuperate your strength!

You will have several medications to take: one to control your diabetes, one to help your blood cells get stronger and another one to help you with heartburns. I will prescribe a sleeping pill that you should take every day, at least at the beginning. Rest is as vital as eating to rebuild your system! You will also have to be very careful not to be in contact with sick people. As much as possible, avoid crowds. Should anything occur, anything at all, you must advise us immediately! We cannot afford to take the slightest chance. During your convalescence, I will see you every two weeks, at least at the beginning, to make sure that all is going well. I think I have said it all and should you have any questions, even if you do not think that it is important, you must call your Protocol nurse. We need to be made aware of the slightest change that occurs. It is really important. Did you understand everything?"

I am shaking like a leaf, I am so excited! I am totally beyond myself! I cannot even find the words to answer him. All I can think of right now is:

'I am going home tomorrow; I cannot believe it, tomorrow! It is incredible! I cannot contain myself! I am so anxious to call all my loved ones and give them the 'super-super' good news. We have been waiting, hoping and praying for this moment to come for such a long time! I cannot believe it has finally arrived!'

It is as though the Doctor can read my mind because after several seconds, he repeats his question. This more or less brings me back down to earth! I look at him with tears in my eyes and say:

"Yes Doctor, I think I understood almost everything you said! You must try to understand; I have been here for already 25 days! I am so anxious and so excited to go home! I do understand and know very well that all this is not finished yet; I still have to take very good care of myself and take it easy. As far as eating goes Doctor, I would not worry too much about all this if I were you! As soon as I am home Peter will take over, he will cook meals that will be easy to eat and very easy to digest. Believe me, he will keep a very close watch on me and make sure that I eat regularly and that I rest well. This Doctor, I can guarantee you!"

He looks at me and says:

"Good luck Madame and take care of yourself! We are all very happy for you! Do you have any questions at this time?"

"No Doctor, not at this time! I do want to take this opportunity to thank you very sincerely for all that you have done for me since the very beginning of this awful and terrible sickness. Please transmit my most sincere thanks to all your colleagues who have given so much of their precious time: 'THANK YOU' from the bottom of my heart!"

I am jubilating! I am so happy! Finally, I am going home! I jump on the phone but too excited, I cannot even dial the number! The good woman next to me comes to my rescue and dials the number for me. As soon as Peter answers, I scream:

"Sweetie, I am coming home! The Doctor is going to sign my release tomorrow! Is this good news or what? Is it not wonderful? I am at the peak of happiness! I can hardly contain myself! Tomorrow, can you imagine? I will finally be home with you tomorrow! It has been so long! Oh Peter, I am shaking, I am so happy! As soon as the Doctor leaves after signing my release tomorrow, I will call you. I hope that you will pick me up right away. I am so anxious to get out of here; I cannot imagine spending one extra second in this room. Can you understand Darling? Please say that you understand! Ah Peter, if only you knew how excited I am to be back home with you every hour of the day, to sleep in a super comfortable bed, to be able to walk around as I please, to be back in my things. I am so anxious to be back in our beautiful love nest!"

He listens patiently, does not interrupt once and finally, when I stop talking, seriously he says:

"Well, you know Cookie, I will have to think about this and organize my agenda in consequence! After all, I am a very busy man you know!"

After hearing this, I scream:
"What? You have to think about it? You have to organize your daily schedule? What on earth is...?"

I hear him laugh at the other end of the line! He says:
"What a question to ask Sweetie! You know very well that I will come and get you with great pleasure! The apartment has been so empty since you have gone! I will be at the hospital even before you can dial the number! I am so anxious to have you here with me day and night! You will see Cookie, everything will be fine! I will see you later and bring you some hot chicken broth. I love you Darling and I can hardly wait until tonight!"

I am simply filled with joy and the lady next to me is very happy for me. I call Lily and Eric and give them the good news. They cry and scream of joy and cannot stop saying that they are so anxious to come and see me and hold me tight. I call René-Luc to give him the good news and the reason why he had to leave the room so abruptly this morning when the Doctor arrived.

After listening to my exclamations without interruption, he says:
"At least I had to leave for a very good reason! I am so happy for you! Finally, your prayers and ours have been answered! You really deserve all this joy after all the suffering you have been through!"

I am so happy and relieved to have all these wonderful people to talk to. I have the impression that it prevents me from going completely out of my mind! Such excitement can drive you out of control...

Shortly after talking with René-Luc, Eric enters the room. We hug, we laugh and we cry! We are completely ecstatic. I cannot stop repeating:

"Do you realize Darling, I am going home tomorrow? I can hardly believe it! It seems too good to be true! If only you knew how much I want to get out of here, get rid of all the tubes hanging on me. I cannot wait to wear something else than this hospital night gown, to be able to put color on my face, wear my wig or a nice little scarf and try to look more like a 'Woman'! Eric, do you have the slightest idea of how happy I am, do you?"

After all this excitement, I am exhausted and I have to sit down. I still cannot stop talking and sweet Eric listens patiently. I can see the joy in his eyes and on his face! He is all smiles and keeps staring at me. After a while, he takes my hands and says:

"Mom, you have to calm down, you are still very weak and you have to be careful. I understand your happiness and you have every right to be this happy! You have to try to calm down a little bit otherwise, you will have a heart attach. We are all elated and also very happy for you!"

I try to calm down and be more relaxed, but it is so difficult! Half an hour later, Lily appears in the door! She too is very excited and there we go again; we hug, we jump, we laugh and we cry all at the same time. Our joy is at its peak! This is sheer madness!!!

We are all so happy and so grateful for all these wonderful moments! The road has been very long and very hard! Thanks to God, the medical core and to my super great team, we made it! I am still alive, not strong but alive! What an accomplishment! What a victory!

My Dear and Great Lord how can we ever thank you enough for giving us all this joy and giving me another chance?

In the meantime, the nurse comes in the room and deposits a tray on my table. To say the truth, no one even noticed it! When she returns to pick it up, I had not even opened it. Actually, I am totally incapable of eating whatsoever right now! My joy, my happiness and my euphoria are sufficient nourishment for the moment! The nurse understands and takes the tray away! Before she passes the door, I promise that I will eat tonight. She looks at me with a nice smile and leaves.

While Lily and I sit on the bed, Eric takes a chair and sits in front of us and we try to stay calm. We talk of different subjects and everything is interesting. I am so thankful to have them both here with me! What a glorious reward!

After the children leave, I lie down and try to rest a little. Impossible, I simply cannot stay in place! I get up and talk with my neighbor.

Around six o'clock that evening, Peter comes in. He takes me in his arms and gives me a big hug. God it feels good!

He looks at me and I cannot help thinking how wonderful it will be to be home together again. To sit side by side on our famous sofa, to hold hands and thank God for all that He has done for us and for all that He gives so generously!

Peter and I walk in the corridor and we cannot stop talking. I tell him all that the Doctor told me this morning, all the warnings, the precautions I have to take and the huge number of medications he will prescribe. After listening to me attentively, he says:
"I do not want you to worry Darling, I will take very good care of you and make sure that you eat and rest well every day. Everything will be fine, I assure you!"

Too soon, we hear on the microphone:
"Visiting hours are over! All visitors are asked to kindly leave."

Sadly, Peter walks me back to the room! We kiss and, before leaving, he says:
"I will see you tomorrow Sweetie and do not worry, I will be here shortly after lunch. You must try to sleep and rest a little bit; you really need the rest after all the excitement!"

144

Although I have mentioned this before, I cannot help reminiscing:

'These last 25 days have been hell for me, for Peter, for my little 'Mine Mines', for Lily and Eric, for René-Luc and for all our friends. Today, the Lord allows us to rejoice! He allows us to dream of our future, whatever the length may be. He is giving me a second chance to life. He gives me more time to be with all the people I love most on this earth. He is also giving me the hope of having better tomorrows. What more can I possibly ask for? After having gone so far down, having almost touched death, how can I even begin to explain the awesome sensation that is within me? It is impossible to find the right words that would explain this extraordinary feeling!'

What a great reward for me to see all these smiling faces, the contentment, the happiness and the brightness that shines in the eyes of my beloved ones. What great victory I have achieved by surviving it all and how sweet it is to go back home tomorrow! I feel that this joy is contagious and I pray the Lord that it lasts and lasts. Deep inside I say:

'Life is so wonderful! How much happier can I be? I feel so privileged!'

Tomorrow is not very far! Peter and the children will not have to come to the hospital every day and return home broken-hearted. I have a feeling that sleep will be scarce for everyone tonight; we are all too excited!

Thursday, last day in the hospital! At six this morning, I am wide-awake; honestly I did not sleep more than five minutes! I could not keep my eyes closed! I sincerely hope that this will be the last morning that I will hear:
"Good morning! It is time for your blood tests!"

Again this morning, I greet the technician with a big smile!

Today I do not need a chair in the washroom; I can stand up to wash myself! As soon as the technician leaves, I start getting ready. Last night, Peter brought my clothes and you have no idea how anxious I am to dress-up, to put makeup on my face, to put on my wig and most of all, to get out of here and breathe some outside air!

I am aware that I have to wait for the Doctor to come by and sign my release before going. Even if the Doctor is aware of how anxious I am to go home, I must not show it too too much.

René-Luc comes by this morning and we go for a walk in the corridor. I tell him:
"I want to take this opportunity to thank you very much for your daily visits, all your encouragement and the great support you have always shown me. I greatly appreciate the friendship we have; we could not have chosen a better moment to rekindle such a worthwhile friendship. If you feel like it, Peter and I would like it very much if you would continue to come over once I am home."

146

After he leaves, I patiently wait for the Doctor to come and finally sign my release! While waiting, the woman next to me sits with me and starts chatting; I guess she wants to help me pass the time.

She talks about her sickness and her family and I listen and try to encourage her as much as possible.

A little before one o'clock, the Doctor finally enters the room! He has checked all my morning tests and all is still very good. After reiterating a few more precautions, he signs my release and says:
"You will be able to leave after two o'clock this afternoon. I wish you the best of luck and do take very good care of yourself!"

After he leaves, I rush in the washroom and get dressed! I put my luggage on the bed and there, everything is ready and so am I! Peter arrives at 1H15 p.m. and takes the luggage to the car. When he returns, we patiently wait for two o'clock.

At two o'clock sharp, with a big smile on our faces, we say 'Goodbye' to everyone and off we go! Finally, I am on my way home! What ecstasy! What happiness! I am alive and I am absolutely and totally happy!

X

Finally, I go home...

When we arrive home, Peter pushes the door wide-open. There in the middle of the dinning table, I can see a huge bouquet of long stem red roses. They are so pretty! As I come closer to smell them, my attention is drawn towards the balconies that are full of geraniums. The morning before my return home, Peter filled the flower boxes with beautiful red geraniums so that I would have nice flowers all summer long.

As I walk around, I find everything so beautiful; I had almost forgotten! I am so happy to be back!

I have not been sleeping very well lately and with all this excitement, all of a sudden, I become very tired and I have to lie down. How good it feels just to be in my bed, in my blankets and on my pillow! It is so comfortable and it feels great! In no time at all, I am gone in la-la-land and I sleep for a couple of hours.

While I am sleeping, Peter unpacks my things and slowly prepares dinner. My first meal at home in such a long time; I do not remember having found Peter's cooking so delicious! Of course, I cannot eat very much, but being home makes it even more succulent! There is also a full pot of my 'miracle soup' already waiting for me! If I ever needed strength, now is the time I need it most! I promise Peter to start eating my soup as soon as tomorrow.

Shortly after dinner, I am still very tired; I have to go back to bed! I am overwhelmed to see how fast I tire and how weak I am. Now I understand why the Doctor was warning me to take all these precautions! I will really have to be very careful!

I honestly thought that being at home in my things would be a lot easier. I thought that I was more resilient than I actually am. I thought that my strength would come back faster. As soon as my head touches the pillow, I am fast asleep. I must say that I find this quite encouraging and I hope that it will help me recover my strength!

This is my first Saturday at home and the first morning that, at six o'clock, I do not hear: "Good morning! It is time for your blood tests!"

After breakfast, Peter and I sit side by side on the sofa and admire our little love nest. It is so good to be back! I cannot find the words to express my happiness!

149

A little later, René-Luc comes for a visit and offers me 12 long-stem yellow roses, what a beautiful bouquet! The three of us sit on the balcony with a cup of coffee and chat while admiring the garden, the wonderful red geraniums and the quiet river. What a view! God this is great!

In the afternoon, Lily, Cassandra and Karl-David come for a visit. They offer me a nice bouquet with two birds of paradise, red, yellow and pink roses, and more. What a nice arrangement, it is very pretty!

As they said:
"We were not allowed to bring you flowers in the hospital because you were in isolation. Now no one can stop us from making sure that you have flowers all around you!"

It is fantastic! I am so happy to see the 'Mine- Mines'. This time, no one can stop me from hugging and kissing them as much as I want, as long as they agree...

That evening, Rick comes over for a visit. It has been quite a while since his last visit. Because of his work, he is often on the road and when he is in town, he tries to see his Father as often as he can. We have a very good time and Peter is always happy to see him. It was a pleasant visit!

As I lie in bed tonight, I cannot help thinking of the beautiful day I had today. It was so good to have all our loved ones around us. I am tired yes, but overjoyed!

In my prayers tonight, I thank God for giving me such a wonderful day; I thank Him for giving me a second chance to life. I also ask Him to watch over Peter and me and over our precious loved ones.

No sooner have I finished my prayer, I fall sound asleep and have beautiful dreams.

I slept very well last night, with the help of the sleeping pills of course. I really feel rested on this beautiful Sunday morning. Peter and I have our breakfast on the balcony; it is a beautiful sunny day.

At the beginning of the afternoon, Eric comes over with his girlfriend and we all chat together. He says:

"I was not able to come over yesterday because I was out of town all day. Mom I am so glad that you are finally home, it is so wonderful! It feels good to see you elsewhere than in a hospital room. I am proud of you Mom and I love you."

"I love you too Darling! Again, thank you very much for all that you have done since the beginning of this awful sickness. You were always so present. And 'YES' I am really happy to finally be back home."

They do not stay very long because Eric notices that I am getting tired. So we chat a little longer and they leave.

It was a very short visit but I was very happy to see them both and we had a good time together.

After they leave, I have no choice but to go and lie down for a little siesta. I am really tired!

When I wake up, Peter is in the kitchen preparing supper and I join him. I am standing in front of the stove watching the hamburger buns when all of a sudden, everything goes black and down I go.

I did not even have time to say or do anything; I simply fell like a rag! Even if Peter is right there close to me, he did not have time to react at all. I fell within a second and I hit the side of the drawer. Thank God I only had a few scratches, nothing serious.

Peter helps me up and brings me to the sofa. We both ask ourselves what on earth could have happened, what caused this? To fall like this for no reason whatsoever, it is quite disturbing.

Needless to say that after falling like this, I did not do a thing for the rest of the evening. As soon as I moved a finger, Peter was right there! This fall really scared us both!

The following morning, at eight o'clock sharp, I call my guardian Angel to inform her of what happened last night. As I start explaining, she stops me saying:
"During your convalescence, you must refer to the auto graft specialist. She will keep your dossier and take charge of you until the end of your convalescence. I will recuperate your dossier afterwards."

I call the auto graft specialist and give her a thorough explanation of what happened to me last night. She listens carefully, asks a few questions and says:

"By what you are telling me, it could very well be that you have had a drastic drop of blood pressure. With all that you have been through lately, it does happen sometimes. You are still very weak and you probably exerted yourself! Rest well for two to three days and things should return to normal. Should it reoccur, you will have to come to the hospital immediately in order to undergo further tests to see what is really going on."

Thank God, it did not happen again! I must say that, during the following three days, Peter was constantly by my side and followed my every move.

My first full week at home passes slowly but surely! I sleep in the morning, in the afternoon and I am back in bed quite early at night. I still tire fast and I am still quite weak! It is as though I have no resistance and no endurance whatsoever!

I join Peter in the kitchen and try to help sometimes; but I have to be very careful and listen to the demands of my body.

Peter checks me all the time and makes sure that I do not overdo it, that I do not stand up too long and most of all, he makes sure that I eat well, that I have my 'miracle soup' every day and that I get all the rest I need.

He often tells me:

"Cookie, I can see when you are hungry and when you become tired; it is as though all the blood disappears from your face and you become very pale."

Towards the end of my first week at home, I start preparing a 'thank you' note for the personnel of the hospital who took such good care of me during my long stay. I absolutely want to send this note to the head-nurse on the 6th floor. We often say that 'writings last forever' and it is very important for me that I do this.

The nurses were so kind and so nice! They really worked hard to help me get out of this ordeal and I want my note to last forever! Peter helps me put it together and once the draft is done; I finalize it!

I already know that Eric is coming over on Friday night and I will ask him to deliver the letter directly to the 6th floor of the hospital.

When Eric arrives on Friday, the three of us sit comfortably on the balcony and chat. Before he leaves, I ask him:

"Darling, would you please do me a little favor? Would you mind depositing this letter at the reception of the 6th floor Ward of the hospital? I really would like it to be hand delivered."

"Of course Mom, it will be my pleasure! I will deliver it tomorrow morning! Do not worry; I will take care of it!"

Now I am satisfied!

We are now in the month of June and the school year is nearly finished! Peter and I already know that we will not be able to have the 'Mine-Mines' this summer, I will not be strong enough. Besides, I had already asked the Doctor who replied:

"I know that you would love to have your grandchildren for a few days this summer, but you must realize that you have just come out of a very difficult period. I honestly do not think that you are strong enough. It has not been long enough since you came out of the hospital and you are still in convalescence. We cannot take any chances now, it would not be wise. I do hope you understand!"

I am very sad to think that they will not come this summer, but I do understand that the Doctor cannot allow this and of course, I know that he is right.

Since my return from the hospital, there has not been one day that we did not have visitors. Lily comes with the 'Mine-Mines'; Eric comes alone and sometimes with his girlfriend, Rick with or without Diane and René-Luc comes by a few times a week.

There are even some neighbors in the condominium that drop by to tell me how worried they were and how hard they prayed for me to get well. Some come to say 'Hello' and bring me flowers! I am so touched by their kindness and concern! The friends also call and are anxious to come and see us!

155

I had asked our friends not to come to the hospital, firstly because of the seriousness of the situation, the isolation and because the Doctor thought it preferable not to have an excess of visitors. Secondly, I would not have been at ease; always in 'that' hospital gown, no makeup and no hair. I could not even endure my wig; not even a scarf on my head. With the family, it was different!

Now that I am back home, I can dress up, put some color on my face and wear my wig. I must say that I feel and look a lot better!

I must admit that we have wonderful friends; not one of them questioned my decision. I appreciated their kindness and their understanding! You know your real friends when they show so much respect!

Two weeks after my release from the hospital, Peter and I go for my first visit with the Oncologist. Once in his office, he looks at me and says:
"I find you quite pale Madame! Are you eating properly and resting well as the Doctor ordered? I still have not received your blood test results but when I do, we will know whether we need to have further tests made."

He examines me thoroughly and after writing down the results of his exam, says:
"If we find anything in the blood tests, we will call you immediately. For the time being, I strongly suggest that you do not go into big crowds and be in contact with sick people.

Even a simple cold could be very harmful for you at this time. If your blood cells are low, it could become very dangerous; your immune system is still very weak. You must make sure to eat well and take a lot of rest. This is very important if you want to recuperate your strength. If you do not hear from us today or tomorrow, I will see you again in two weeks. By then, we will know more with the results of the blood tests. The nurse will schedule your next appointment."

When we come home, I have to go and lie down, I am exhausted! Imagine a simple little trip to the hospital and I am bushed, I am not 'super woman'. I do hope to recuperate my strength as soon as possible!

In the afternoon, the auto graft specialist calls and says:
"The Doctor has received the results of your blood tests and he says that your red blood cells are low and you are a little anemic. Your potassium level is also low and the Doctor has prescribed a medication to help regulate your potassium. If you could give me the telephone number of your pharmacy, I will order them for you. It would be good if you could pick them up as soon as possible because the Doctor did say that you should start taking them immediately. Be very careful not to find yourself in a crowd and you must absolutely avoid being in contact with sick people. Take good care of yourself!"

After talking to Peter about my conversation with the auto graft specialist and mentioning what she said about the anemia, Peter decides to make my 'miracle soup' again. I try to eat the soup twice a day, but since we are in summer and that it is very warm, I find it hard to eat a heavy soup like this.   To encourage me, Peter decides to have some soup with me!

In the month following our last visit to the Oncologist, our only outings are to see the Doctor and go for my blood tests.

Lily, Eric and René-Luc come to visit us regularly, which of course if very good for our moral. Rick comes more often now that I am home.   His visits are good for Peter: they encourage him very much!

One day, during one of Eric's visit, as we are sitting on the balcony and chatting, all of a sudden he says:

"Mom, do you remember that terrible Friday after the auto graft when you were feeling so bad? I was coming to see you and on the way, I met your Doctor in the hallway. I stopped and asked him how you were really doing. After listening to him until he stopped talking, I entered your room. When I saw you lying there, so pale with all those bags of medication hanging on you, Mom, I just could not move. It was as though I had been 'struck' by lightning. I cried so hard and could not take my eyes off of you. I do not know how long I stood there…

I was so afraid of losing you and I was scared that you would not pull through this ordeal. I was praying so hard for a miracle that would cure you. Mom, do you realize how good it is to see you sitting here with me, talking and laughing, and alive? I thank you so much for fighting that hard and I am so very proud of you! I love you Mom!"

I am so moved that I cannot even speak! Eric and I sit there holding hands and tears roll down our cheeks. I do not know how long we stayed like this without even talking, but after a while, Eric stands up and takes me in his arms. He gives me a big hug and leaves!

Between the visits, I try to rest as much as I can and Peter makes sure that I eat well. Of course, we also make sure that all our visitors are in very good health. Everyone is aware of the danger I am in right now because of my low red blood cells.

At my mid-August visit with the Oncology specialist and after he finishes his exam, I ask him:

"We are now in the middle of August and so far, I honestly have been very good! I was wondering if you would agree to let us take the 'Mine-Mines', for a few days before they go back to school in September?"

He does not answer right away! He continues writing in my dossier that is becoming thicker and thicker... He turns to my guardian Angel and asks:

"Have you received the results of her last blood tests?"

I had already taken the blood tests two days before my visit; therefore, I knew that the results would be in. My guardian Angel hands him the sheet of paper containing the results and he exams them closely. After, and only after, he looks at me and says:

"The exam I made is good and so are your blood tests. You are not very strong yet and you must continue to be very careful and not exert yourself. You have to be sure that the children have no cold, no virus or anything else. Therefore, if you accept all these conditions, then for a few days only, I have no objections!"

The Doctor, my guardian Angel and Peter look at me and apparently my entire face illuminated like a Xmas tree. I look at the Doctor and with a huge smile, I say:

"Doctor, I accept all your conditions with great pleasure! I will make sure with my daughter Lily that they are both in very good health. I promise that I will not exert myself and that I will continue taking very good care of myself. Besides, Peter takes full charge of our meals, the children set the table and clean it after the meal and my little Cassandra always washes the dishes; she pretends that she enjoys doing it. You know, it will be awesome to have these little Sweethearts with us even for only a few days. They are such a good therapy for me!"

Peter looks at the Doctor and says:
"Do not worry too much Doctor! I will be there all the time and make sure that she does not tire and that everything goes well!"

We shake hands with the Doctor and thank him very much!

No sooner am I sitting in the car, I call Lily and say:
"Hello Darling, how are you? I saw the Doctor this morning, he is satisfied with the exam, and the blood tests are good. I asked him if we could take the children for a few days before they go back to school and he agreed. Do you think the children would accept to come over for a few days? I would like that so much! We would go to the pool, play cards and their society games that they like so much. We have so much fun when we are all together! What do you say Darling, will you ask them? Of course, you have to make sure that they are in very good health!"

Lily calls fifteen minutes later and says:
"Mom, the children are very excited and anxious to go over for a few days. Do not worry Mom; they are in very good health! We will bring them over Wednesday after work and pick them up around lunchtime on Saturday. Is this convenient for you? Should you become tired, you promise to call me right away!"

"Yes, Yes, I promise! I cannot wait until Wednesday! Thank you Darling!"

Finally Wednesday and the kids arrive! We are so happy to see them! We go to the pool, play cards and talk about everything with them; they are so interesting to listen too!

We have so much fun with these two wonderful children; we are like real kids ourselves. Peter is more than happy to concoct all the goodies the kids love best. On Friday night, Peter prepares everything for our 'traditional' dinner feast. What a joyful and beautiful evening we have!

I cannot believe that it is already Saturday! It is too soon! When Lily and Marc-André arrive we gather around the table and eat Peter's delicious pancakes. It is great to be all together! They leave at three p.m. and we find ourselves alone again!

All of a sudden, the house is so empty! It is incredible how the presence of these two 'Mine-Mines' changes the atmosphere. Even though we only had them for a few days, it was really worth it! I enjoyed them to the fullest and what a great therapy for me!

We return to our little routine! Their short visit really lifted me up!

After the 'Mine-Mines' visit, I have another meeting with the Oncologist. After a meticulous exam, he asks that I go for a Gallium scan and a cardiac ultrasound.

On the following visit, at the end of August, the Doctor had received all the results of the tests and says:

"In general, the exams are good, but we have detected a spot on your right hip. For the moment, we cannot say whether it is in repair or if it is lymphoma. Therefore, I would like you to go for a PET scan! This exam is a lot more precise and it should help us see more clearly. I also would like you to meet the Cardiologist to verify your heart. Your guardian Angel will make all the appointments and call you back with the details."

Eric is with Peter and me for this visit and after listening carefully to the Doctor, the three of us are very disappointed that I have more tests to take. Is it simply a spot or is there something in the wind? One thing is sure: I am very anxious to get the results...

During the auto graft, the Oncologist had informed Lily and Eric that:
"Should the sickness recur, it would be a very bad sign and the sickness could progress very rapidly. Your Mother would still be too weak to fight this new sickness. It would not be long before she would become very ill and maybe even worse..."

Of course, the Doctor had not mentioned any of this to Peter nor I! He probably did not want to discourage us!

When the Oncologist asks for more tests, Eric turns very pale. He remembers what the Doctor had said during the auto graft. He is afraid that the sickness is back which makes him more anxious to get the results.

At that precise moment, I had not noticed that Eric's face had changed. It is only a little while later when I recalled the visit that I remembered that effectively Eric had become tense and very pale at the announce of the new tests prescribed by the Doctor.

Two days after my visit with the Oncologist, my guardian Angel calls back with the dates and times of the PET scan and the visit with the Cardiologist. She adds:

"As soon as we receive all the results of the tests, I will call you back and give you an appointment date for your next visit with the Oncologist."

The following week we meet the Cardiologist. As soon as we are seated in his office, he asks:

"Have you had heart pains in your chest? Do you feel tightness around the heart? Did you have to take any nitroglycerine pills since your last visit?"

"I took nitroglycerine twice since I was here last! The first time it happened was when I woke up one morning; I had not made any efforts at all, not even a fast move, absolutely nothing. Yet I had this pain in my chest and I decided to put a nitroglycerine pill under my tongue. A few minutes later, the pain was gone! The second time; I was sitting very quietly and I was knitting when I felt a similar pain to my heart. Without even getting up, I asked Peter to bring me a nitroglycerine pill.

As the first time, after a few minutes, the pain was gone completely. Those are the only two times that I felt this kind of pain in my chest and that I took a nitroglycerine pill. Tell me Doctor, why are you asking me all these questions? Have you discovered something abnormal? I honestly hope not!"

"At your last cardiac ultrasound, we discovered that you had water in the pericardium area (that is the conical membranous sac enveloping the heart in vertebrates). This could have been caused by the massive chemotherapy that you had received during the auto graft of the bone marrow. Whatever the reason was, we must follow this very closely and make sure that it does not get worse. We will know more in a few more weeks."

During the months of September and October, Peter and I start going out a little more. We go and have lunch with Lily; go to restaurants, sometimes with Eric, other times with Rick. We even risk ourselves and go to the Shopping Centre to walk around a little and look at the new fashions in the stores. Unfortunately, I cannot walk very long because I still tire quickly.

For my birthday in October, Peter and I decide to go dancing with Andrée and Renald. They are both very happy to see that I feel strong enough to come out. We do not dance very much but the simple fact of dressing up is very good for both our morals.

It has been quite a long time since we last went dancing at our favorite dance Hall and it feels very good to see everyone. It goes without saying that the people have heard of our mishaps! Several friends come to see us and say:

"How are you doing Madame and how are you Sir? It has been so long since we have seen you last and it is nice to see you both!"

It feels so good to see everyone! I have the impression I am reborn, I feel alive again! Peter is so proud of me and very happy to see all the people coming to greet us. What a wonderful evening!

We go downtown and have lunch with Eric. Another time, we have lunch with Lily! It is paradise on earth to go out and have a normal life.

It is so fantastic to feel good enough and be able to go where we want, when we want! Even more so, what a great feeling to be part of this wonderful world! I appreciate each breath that I take, every moment that I spend with my children and my beloved grandchildren and of course; all the precious time that I have with my dear Peter.

For my anniversary weekend, the children organize a special dinner. We are all invited at Eric's place and René-Luc is there. I am received with gorgeous flowers and many hugs. I am so happy! What a super time I have with all my loved ones!

I have to say that it is an amazing therapy for me when, in only one evening, I can almost forget all the recent hardships we have been through.

Every morning when I open my eyes I feel blessed and privileged to be offered the precious gift of life. God gives me a new breath, a new day and so many wonderful things to live for! Oh! How I thank Him!

A few days after my anniversary, the hospital calls and finally they give me the time and date of the PET ultrasound. Because I will be undergoing the exam only two days before my next visit with the Oncologist, I have no idea if the results will come in on time. I do hope so!

The morning of the PET scan, Peter and I arrive at the hospital at 10H30 a.m. He drops me off in front of the hospital and goes and parks the car. When he joins me, he offers me a beautiful bouquet of gladioluses.

Sweet Peter, he knows that I am extremely nervous! I am claustrophobic and when I think that I will be trapped in a huge tube for several minutes, I panic and I have goose bumps. Peter really does all he can to make things easier on me. I appreciate his every effort!

Finally at 14H25 p.m., the nurse calls me and brings me to the room for the exam; it lasts more than one hour. I can only say that for the claustrophobic that I am; one hour in that tube appears like an eternity...

We leave the hospital way passed four o'clock! When we arrive to the car, I find twelve beautiful red roses sitting on my seat. Dear Peter, he really thinks of the most beautiful things to make my life more joyful! How I thank God for having put this wonderful man on my road!

You might find that all these annotations are quite simple or even ridiculous! Believe me, when you go through so much suffering, so much worrying, anguish and stress, that you touch death so closely, the smallest kindness and the simplest tender gesture count.

I absorb every little joy and appreciate it to the fullest! Take advantage of everything that your surrounding offers you and does for you. Everything helps; it is positive and most important; it keeps your moral up high!

XI

Incurable...

As previously scheduled, two days after the PET ultrasound, December 9th, 2003 Eric, Peter and I go to the Doctor's office for the results. Needless to say that we are all stressed and very nervous...

As in February 2003 - when the Doctor did not even take the time to examine me - he is very serious. He invites us to sit and as usual, goes straight to the point saying:

"Madame, we have received the results of your tests. They show that the sickness has significantly regressed since the auto graft of the bone marrow. Unfortunately, we have depicted some new sickness."

Eric, Peter and I are completely shattered and awe-struck! We understood what the Doctor said, but it seems so impossible, we simply do not want to believe one word of it. Of course, we know that the results are real, but it does not want to sink in!

I look at the Doctor and have the impression I am looking at a total stranger! I try my hardest not to let the tears fall, unfortunately this time I cannot hold them back and they roll non-stop down my face. I make a tremendous effort to regroup myself and finally ask the Doctor:

"How can this be possible? How can the cancer come back so fast? Is it still curable?"

The Doctor understands that we are actually in a state of choc. He can easily see the discouragement on our faces. We have just come out of the auto graft; I am still in my convalescence period. I know that he knows all this and yet...

Down deep inside I cannot help thinking and asking myself:

'Have we done all this for nothing; simply to arrive to this point? I cannot believe that, not after all the suffering, after working so hard to come out of this torturous sickness. After having fought so hard! No, I do not want to believe it, it cannot be true! It is impossible!'

After leaving us to our reflections for a few minutes, the Doctor interrupts our thoughts and says:

"There are still several medications that we can give you to slow down the progression. There are also other medications that could help calm the pain. We can still do an awful lot for you! You have to hang on and not give up! Do not let discouragement take over!"

170

"Are you saying that we are back to last February when you offered us those two options? Given that I have already used the option of the auto graft of the bone marrow, the only one left is the 18 to 24 months of survival! Is this what you are trying to make us understand?"

I know that I am being sarcastic and most of all I know very well that this is not the Doctor's fault. But it hurts so badly! I am so frightened! I simply cannot help myself; it is as though I too want to hurt back!

All the same, God knows that my poor Doctor does not deserve this sarcasm! I know that it is not right to talk this way but I cannot help myself, I hurt too much inside...

The Doctor looks at me and gently says: "I understand how hard this must be for all of you to receive such bad news. I know you are hurting and that you are very scared. I am very well placed to know how much you suffered and how hard you fought. I can assure you that I will do my utmost best to help you as much as I can. Should you need moral support, I could refer you to a good psychologist who will help you and yours get through this ordeal."

The three of us are crying and Eric, who has not said one word since the beginning, looks at the Doctor and asks:
"Do you have any idea of how long we have, Doctor?"

I look at Eric and cry out:
"Oh my God, I most certainly do not want to hear anything on this subject! It will soon be Xmas and please do not talk about it. Please Eric; I do not want to know!"

The Doctor looks at Eric and says:
"Even if I wanted to give you an answer, it is completely impossible! No one really has an answer for that question. No patient reacts the same way with such an awful sickness and I honestly cannot give you a satisfying answer!"

I look at the Doctor and say:
"Thank you for the moral support offer! To begin with, I think that we need to digest what you have told us before anything else. As we so often say:
'Time heals!'
We all need time to assimilate such disturbing news! Should we need moral support at a later time, I will call you and maybe then could you schedule a visit for us. Is that all right with you Doctor?"
"Yes Madame, it is fine!"

We thank him and leave.

In the elevator, no one speaks! Once on the ground floor, Peter says:
"Sweetie, wait here with Eric while I go and get the car!"

Eric takes me in his arms and holds me real tight! He is trying so hard not to burst out in tears. After staying like this for a little while, he says:

172

"Mom, is there something special that you would like to do? Somewhere special you would like to visit: Puerto Rico, Mexico, the Dominican Republic... I know that you have never been to those places. Maybe you would prefer to go elsewhere. Wherever you want Mom! You know, I could easily take two weeks off and we could leave together, the two of us. What do you say Mom?"

We must not forget what the Doctor had told Lily and Eric during my auto graft of the bone marrow to the effect that should the sickness recur, it could go very fast. They should prepare themselves for the worse! Eric is thinking of these words and this is why he wants to offer me the moon and the stars.

I look at him and his cheeks are soaked with tears. My poor Sweetheart, his pain is so great! I cry and I hurt for him, for Peter who wants me to beat this sickness so badly, for Lily and René-Luc who still are not aware of the bad news. My poor little 'Mine-Mines', how will they react to all this? My sweet little ones, they are still so young!

All this suffering and so close to Christmas! What a '**gift**' I am giving them! I love them so much and yet, it is because of me that they suffer so! I know that it is not directly my fault; God knows I did all I possibly could to get better! I fought like a lioness! Nevertheless, I am still the one causing all this pain; I hurt so badly for them!

173

Very sadly and always looking at Eric, I say:

"It is really nice of you Darling to think of this in such trying times! You have no idea how happy you make me! You know Eric; I honestly think that we must regain control of this entire situation. As I said to the Doctor, we must try to digest and assimilate all that has happened. We cannot simply run away from it! Even if we tried our hardest, we cannot run away from ourselves. Besides, it would not change a thing; the sickness would still be there. And the others, what about them: Lily, the 'Mine-Mines' and your Father? They too will suffer when they hear the terrible news! What about my Dear Peter, who has been by my side 24 hours a day since the very beginning, have you thought of him? What would become of him if we left him alone, especially now? No Darling, this is not the time to flee! To the contrary, we must stay all together and try to help one another as much as we possibly can. We must encourage each other and most of all, we must stay strong."

"I understand what you are saying Mom and it makes sense! I only want you to be happy, to see you laugh again and most of all that you do not suffer anymore. I am ready to do anything to see you happy, even if it is only for a few weeks! Do you understand Mom? Can you understand how difficult is it for me to see you suffer like this?"

"Of course I understand Darling and I thank you very much! We would all like to erase everything that was said this morning, but facts are facts and we must face the reality. If there would exist the slightest hope, the slightest way to go ahead as though nothing had happened; believe me Sweetheart, I would be the first one to go forward! This is not over yet, I still have the very difficult task of calling your sister to give her the terribly bad news. This is going to be another excruciating moment! Poor Lily, she will have the horrible task of informing the 'Mine-Mines'. They too are going to hurt badly when they learn about it and just before Xmas... Believe me Darling; I am really not looking forward to this! I do not want to call her at the office with such bad news, I am sure she could not stand it. I will wait until tonight and call her at home."

"Mom, I could go over there tonight and inform her. At least it would be one less terrible moment for you! Do you agree?"

"That is very generous of you Sweetie! I want to tell her myself because, from the beginning of the sickness, I promised to keep you both informed on everything that happens, whether good or bad. Today, you are here with us and you learned about this at the same time we did. Unfortunately, Lily could not be here and I prefer to call her myself. I hope that you can understand!"

"Of course I understand Mom!"

He gives me a big hug and walks me to the car. After such a deceiving morning, he has to go back to work! I can only imagine what kind of afternoon he went through!

Peter and I hardly talk on the way back home. We are totally anchored in our deepest thoughts!

During the last few days, I constantly kept thinking that there might be a recurrence of the sickness; I cannot explain why! However, when the Doctor confirmed my worse nightmare, the choc was terrible for all of us.

As long as we think that, it MIGHT happen, it is not so bad! But when they confirm it, well that is a completely different story. It is like receiving a whiplash! Now I have to face this defeating situation! We all have to face it and believe me; it will not be an easy task for no one!

Once inside the condominium, Peter takes me in his arms and we both cry our eyes out! I could not say how long we stood there; it seemed like an eternity… After we calm down, we sit on the sofa (this sofa has seen a lot since its arrival) and without pronouncing one single word; we try to gather our strength! Slowly we start reliving the matinee we had! All of a sudden we realize that it is dark outside and that neither one of us had lunch nor dinner. We simply stayed there and talked, always coming back to the same question:
'Will I ever be free from this sickness?'

Out of nowhere, the phone rings and it brings us back down to earth! Like a robot, I answer!

What a wake-up when I hear Lily's voice on the phone:

"Good evening Mom! Eric called and asked how I was and if I needed him to come over! When he realized that I knew nothing about your visit to the Doctor's this morning, he asked if you had called me:

'No, why are you asking me this?'

He simply replied:

'You should call her right away!'

Why did you not call me Mom? You always call me, why not this time?"

"I am so sorry Darling! I did not want to call you at the office to give you the results of my visit with the Doctor this morning; I knew that it would be too hard for you. I was going to call you at home this evening to inform you. When Peter and I came home, we both cried a lot! After a long while, we started to talk and we have just now realized that it is night! To tell you the truth Darling, you took us out of our lethargic state when we heard the phone ring. What did Eric tell you exactly?"

"He mentioned a few things but said that you wanted to tell me yourself."

I give her all the details of our morning visit! We both cry and stay on the phone for over one hour. I do my utmost best to answer all her questions!

I honestly think that the fact of having talked on the phone for so long helped us both a great deal!

I know that when Peter and I talked this afternoon, it really did us a lot of good. At least it calmed us a little!

So I tell her:

"You know Darling; we cannot change what has happened today. We have to try our best to accept this new situation! I am convinced that we should all talk about this as much as possible! We must not keep anything inside! We have to ask all the questions that cross our mind; maybe then will we be able to start dealing with all this. We must try, even harder than ever, to live each day that God is willing to give us to the fullest, not waste one second and take out of life everything that we possibly can. For the moment, we are affected only morally; so far I am not suffering physically, thank God! I am still in possession of all my faculties, at least I hope so (we both laugh)! As long as I do not have physical pain, we owe ourselves to embrace life with all our might! We must do our best to take advantage of the festive activities as much as we can. Think of the little 'Mine-Mines' for whom Christmas is still so important! Let us celebrate and enjoy every moment of this glorious season! What do you say Darling?"

No answer! I know that she is crying and that she cannot speak; I continue:

"I understand Sweetheart! If only you knew how hard it is for me to give you such sad news, especially when we are so close to Christmas! I know how afflicting and difficult it can be to have to accept all the highs and lows of this horrible sickness. I also know that we all need time to assimilate and digest all this! Try to rest now! I honestly hope that you will feel a little better tomorrow morning. I will hang up now Darling! Tomorrow, if you are up to it, we can talk again for as long as you want. You know Lily, talking is really the best thing we can do in such a devastating situation. I love you Darling and I am here for you at every hour of the day or night! If you cannot sleep and you feel like talking, please do not hesitate to call me. As I just said, at any time, I will answer you! I love you my Lily and take good care of yourself."

After the call, I join Peter on the sofa and we continue talking! I do not remember what time it was when we went to bed that night; I only remember that Peter held me in his arms and that I cried most of the night. In early morning when I say my prayers, I ask God to forgive me. I confess my discouragement! Yes, I am totally discouraged...

I honestly ask myself: where will I find the strength to continue fighting? I feel so empty; I cannot believe all that is happening! I have no resistance, no will power, nothing left! I even ask myself:

179

'Why am I doing all this? Why should I fight with all my might if it is to be crushed over and over again? I am completely at the end of my rope; I cannot endure anymore...'

It took a very long time for me to fall asleep after my prayers. When I finally doze off, I have very terrifying nightmares! I am completely down in the dumps, I have no courage, no strength left and I seem to lose my will power to continue fighting this awful sickness. I am completely warned-out!

I am still in Peter's arms and I ask God to please prevent him from reading my mind and see all the negative thoughts that go through my head right now.

On the other hand, I sincerely thank the good Lord for having placed Peter on my path; for having given me such wonderful and loving children and grand children! Without even one of them, I can assure you that I would no longer be a part of this world to share with you these episodes of my life!

Sleep was very scarce last night and at nine a.m., René-Luc calls:
"Good morning, how are you feeling? Eric called this morning and told me about your visit to the Doctor. Are you able to talk about it a little bit?"

I am crying, as a matter of fact I am chocking and I simply cannot talk! Patiently, he waits; he knows that I am crying. I do my best to gather myself and finally say:

"I am sorry René-Luc; I cannot talk about this right now! It hurts too much and it is still too fresh! Please, try to understand and give me more time to digest all this and pull myself together. I promise to call you a little later, but it is impossible right now!"

"I understand! It is a very big choc for all of us! I want you to know that if there is anything I can do for you or for Peter, please do not hesitate, anything at all! Would you agree if I came for a visit over the weekend? I promise to call you beforehand!"

"Yes, I think it will be preferable to wait until the weekend and thanks for understanding!"

In the afternoon, Eric calls. He makes tremendous efforts to have a normal voice, but his voice trembles when he says:

"Mom, it is Dad's birthday on Sunday and I thought it could be a great idea if we all got together for a brunch. Lily, Marc-André and the 'Mine-Mines' will be here! Do you think that you and Peter will be able to come? We would all be together; it would be nice, would it not? Will you come?"

What can I say? I would really like to berry myself in a big whole somewhere and let everyone forget me, let them stop hurting because of me! Dear God, I beg of you, please help me; give me the strength to continue!

I have to respect my own saying: whether we like it or not, life does go on! I hope that I will feel better by Sunday!

Besides, what is more important in life than to be surrounded by our family; to be together especially in trying moments like these? We could all have a good cry and afterwards, why not have fun and celebrate! I hardly hear myself saying:

"Darling, you know very well that it is always a great pleasure for us to be with all of you. I know that you are doing this to help us and distract us from all that is happening. Believe me Sweetheart, I greatly appreciate everything you do and I thank you very much for the invitation."

After three days, we start feeling a little better! Eric comes by every day this week and we talk a lot. Lily calls every night and we spend hours on the phone. She is very anxious to come over to see me on Saturday, be close to me and hold me in her arms.

Oh, how I am anxious to hold her in my arms and have her close to me!

As understood, Saturday morning René-Luc calls and asks if he can come over. I feel a little better this morning and I accept.

He arrives an hour later and offers me a dozen of beautiful roses! We hug, we cry and we talk! I do my utmost best to follow the conversation and not to let the commotion inside me come out. I laugh and talk and put on the whole works to show them that I am still very strong. But my God, how bad I hurt inside, it is intolerable!

182

I try to convince myself that we will be able to continue to hang in there like we have done since December 27th, 2001 when I was diagnosed; but honestly I have big doubts that it will be possible...

We are now in December 2003! I am still alive and whatever happens tomorrow or the days after, today I live! I will try my best to take out of life all that it offers!

In the afternoon, Lily comes over! She arrives alone because she really needed to have me all to herself. She offers me a gorgeous bouquet of flowers and puts them in a vase. As she sits next to me, she throws herself in my arms and cries, she says:

"Mom, if only you knew how long I have been waiting for this moment! I am so sorry that I was not able be with you for your visit to the Doctors. I really tried my best to get the day off, but there were two meetings and I was alone in the office to take the calls and receive the people. I absolutely could not liberate myself and I feel so bad about the whole thing. Oh Mom, what I would have given to be with all of you!"

"It must have been very hard on you Darling! However, you know Lily; we cannot always do what we want in life! I am very happy that you are here with me now! After giving it some serious thought, I have concluded that today is today and let tomorrow take care of tomorrow! What do you think of that?"

We sit there side by side for hours and we talk! This is very good therapy for both of us and it helps a great deal! What a constructive and positive visit!

On Sunday morning, Peter and I go off to Eric's brunch to celebrate René-Luc's birthday! Lily, Marc-André, the 'Mine-Mines' and René-Luc are already there.

Peter and I bought a bottle of Champagne to offer to René-Luc for his birthday! He is surprised but very happy! We hug and kiss and reunite around the table for a superb meal! The 'Mine-Mines' are very happy to see us and thank God, they do not ask too many questions concerning the sickness.

It is true that Lily always answers all their questions when they ask! They both stay very close to me and hold my hand! It feels so good to have them close! What great satisfaction they bring me! I hang on to their little hands with all the power left in me!

Children are always so natural and sincere! They may not be able to put all their feelings into words; but they have their own little ways of expressing them! The food at the brunch is sumptuous as usual and for a while, the fact of being surrounded by all my loved ones gives me the courage and the hope that I cannot seem to find within myself.

When we return home, I must admit that Peter is feeling much better and I am happy for him.

Slowly and with no enthusiasm at all, Peter and I begin our Xmas shopping. To say the truth, we find it very hard and we cannot seem to find anything appealing. Even the Xmas decorations in the stores, that usually touch me very much, leave me totally indifferent this year.

But Xmas is getting closer and closer and we actually have no choice to do our shopping now whether or not we feel like it!

The following Tuesday while we are having lunch, Peter says:

"Cookie, what would you say to the idea of going out for a nice car ride this afternoon! It is such a beautiful sunny day and it would do us both a lot of good!"

"Sweetie, I honestly do not feel like going out! Besides, where do you want to go?"

"Nowhere special; it is simply to go for a drive! Come on, say yes; it would be good for us!"

He takes the direction to go downtown! I know that it is too late to have lunch with Eric! I am still wondering where on earth he is taking me when suddenly, he stops the car.

I look around and at the corner; there is a street full of stores. I say to myself:

'He must have found my Christmas gift on this street and now he wants to know if it will please me...'

I am not completely in the wrong because, on the other side of the street, there is a jewelry store.

As we enter, Peter takes my arm and guides me to the ring counter! He asks the sales lady to show us the rings!

I have such great pleasure trying them on one after the other! All of a sudden, my eyes are attracted by one ring in particular! Peter looks in the same direction and sees it. He takes the ring and passes it on my ring finger.

It is simply magnificent and of course, it fits me like a glove! I cannot get over it, it is so beautiful!

Peter looks at the sales lady and smilingly says:
"Well, I guess our choice has been made! This seems to be the one."

The woman replies:
"You both have a very good taste! The ring is wonderful on your finger. I can only offer you my most sincere congratulations!"

Peter goes with the sales woman to finalize the transaction while I stand there like a zombie! I simply cannot stop admiring the ring; it dazzles me!

To say the truth, I still do not understand what has happened; all I seem to be able to think about is the ring. When Peter joins me, he says:
"Cookie, we can leave now!"

I look at him and I still do not know what to do exactly! Seeing my hesitation, he takes me by the arm and guides me towards the door. I have the ring on my finger…

We go back to the car and once we are both comfortably sitting down and still starring at the ring on my finger, I turn towards Peter and ask him:

"Sweetie what does all this mean? What has happened in there? Why did you do this? I still do not understand! Could you please tell me what is going on?"

With his tender smile, he looks at me straight in the eyes, takes my hand and very softly says:

"Darling, I think that you deserve an exceptional gift with everything that is happening in our lives right now! I really wanted to do this! I want to see you happy, to see you smile again. I want to show you how proud I am of you! I love you Sweetheart! The ring is a very small proof of my love! It is my gift of appreciation, my gift of love, my Xmas gift! Call it whatever you want, I simply want to see you happy! Are you happy?"

"What woman would not be, with such a jewel? It is so beautiful! It is magnificent! I thank you from the bottom of my heart and I love you! You know Sweetie, with everything that you have been doing for me since the beginning of this horrible and terrifying sickness, the ring was absolutely not necessary! You do know this!"

"Yes Darling, I know very well that it was not a necessity! As I said; I really wanted to do this and I am very glad that I did!"

This beautiful ring has never left my finger since Peter put it on! I even consider it as my 'engagement ring'.

The following Saturday, we go dancing with our friends Andrée and Renald. We have a wonderful evening! We really try hard to improve each day the Lord offers us and keep as busy as we possibly can.

On Xmas Eve, René-Luc comes over and has breakfast with us. Again, he offers me twelve beautiful peach roses. They are superb! He says:

"I cannot be at Lily's Xmas Eve party tonight and I wanted to come and wish you both a very Merry Xmas. Health, health and more health; this is the utmost I can wish for you. Enjoy the Xmas season to the fullest!"

We thank him sincerely for his wishes and offer him our best wishes for the Xmas season. We greatly appreciate his visit!

After he leaves, Peter and I decide to take a little siesta. As every Xmas Eve parties, the evening will probably go on until the wee hours and we want to be in good shape for the party. As I said before, we really want to enjoy every moment we spend with the children and the grandchildren.

It goes without saying that our hearts are not in a celebrating mood and that I do not really feel like being with anyone. I hurt so badly, the pain does not want to go away! My discouragement is not getting any better either!

For the children and the 'Mine-Mines' and of course for Peter, I must force myself to keep a smile on my face. I want to show them that I am still strong. Dear God, I beg of you, please help me!

When we get to Lily's, Eric and Marc-André's family are there. They are all very happy to see us and greet us warmly.

After the champagne toast, we gather around the beautifully decorated table and enjoy a succulent meal.

We all try very hard to keep our spirits high and have fun! It is so nice to spend this precious time all together!

A little before midnight, the children can no longer wait, they want their presents!

Lily invites us around the Xmas tree and acting as 'Mama Clause', distributes the gifts. Of course, she gives one to each child to quiet them down. They have already been very good to wait this long!

It is so wonderful to see the expressions on their little faces when they discover their present. We cannot help but smile when we see so much joy and happiness!

Children have magic powers; their smile is contagious! To see them so overwhelmed is such a great reward for me!

We have a wonderful time at Lily's place! They all found my ring gorgeous and are very happy for both of us! Peter is very proud of their compliments.

189

For the past eleven years, Peter and I have always celebrated Xmas day only the two of us. Peter prepares a delicious meal and we accompany the meal with our preferred champagne. I dress-up the table nicely and we enjoy soft music!

It is going to be different this year! Because René-Luc could not make it for Lily's Xmas Eve party, he invited all of us for a Xmas dinner at his place.

This time, the Xmas presents will be given before dinner, so the children will not have to wait and suffer too long.

After the children receive their gifts and after all their exclamations; we gather around the table and enjoy a great meal.

For a few hours, we are all reunited, happy and joyful and we try not to think of our pain. Tomorrow is another day...

We have to admit that God acts in mysterious ways sometimes! Today was another proof! We spent another wonderful day with our loved ones.

The day after Xmas, Rick and Diane come over for breakfast. We all exchange gifts and find ourselves around a table once more. We savor a wonderful meal, chat, laugh and once again, have a beautiful day.

Christmas is really a joyful holiday and creates several outings and happy events! To date, we have had several celebrations, a lot of fun and beautiful gifts!

All these cheerful outings and reunions are a big help for both of us and allow us to temporarily forget our fears and pains.

The Sunday after Xmas, celebrations continue and Lily, Marc-André, the 'Mine-Mines, Eric and René-Luc come over for Peter's pancakes. They love his pancakes and always ask for more!

After the meal, Cassandra and Karl-David clean up the table and wash the dishes. They grow so fast! We stay seated at the table and continue chatting and sipping our coffee!

It is always a great joy for me every time I am with my 'Mine-Mines'. I never get tired and I am so proud of them! I am overwhelmed to still be alive to be able to enjoy them and see them grow. I suppose that it is normal for a Mamie to be so taken by her little Darlings and to want to have them around her as often as she possibly can.

Since my last visit to the Oncologist, it seems that I am constantly looking for all kinds of ways to keep busy in the hope that I will not think of my sickness as much. Each time we have an outing, every time I am surrounded by my children or my grandchildren, I never seem to get enough and they become my drug. I must admit that, as a therapy, I could not find a better one!

After they leave, Peter and I decide to go dancing tonight. Why not? After all, it is the Holiday season!

Dancing is very good! The crowd, the loud music, the atmosphere, everything helps. Even if it is only for a few hours, it is really worth it! Have I not already said that we must hang on to anything and everything?

We meet friends and they congratulate me for my new (pixie) hair do. It is the first time I go out without my wig! I must say that their compliments really touched me and made me very happy!

Finally, the last day of 2003! Whether we like it or not, time does flies! Marc-André and the 'Mine-Mines' come to see us but, Lily is not with them because she is working today. Marc-André came over to install the Internet on Peter's new computer.

Not even twenty minutes later, Eric rings the doorbell! He goes out on the balcony and barbecues the steaks. What a wonderful meal! What is better than to be surrounded by our loved ones especially on the last day of such a disastrous year?

It would have been perfect if Lily could have been here! But as they say:
"Nothing is ever perfect on this earth!"

After they leave, Peter and I take a long nap after which we get ready to celebrate New Years Eve at our dance Hall!

XII

Good riddance to 2003...

This is already the eleventh year that Peter and I met here at the dance Hall 'Le Rendez-vous'. To date, we have never missed one New Year's Eve celebration!

We reserved our tickets with Andrée and Renald in order to be seated together. This is the fourth consecutive year that the four of us will greet the New Year.

We have so much fun! They distribute hats, flutes and serpentines. They have balloons on every table. The dance Hall is totally decorated with tinsel garlands and more... The atmosphere is simply electrifying!

We start getting ready for the party at seven p.m. When we arrive at the dance Hall, Andrée and Renald are already there, the music is playing and the dance floor is full.

We talk; I should say we scream to hear one another. At 11 o'clock, they start serving the delicious meal.

For New Year's Eve dinner, they have a special menu! It consists of: soup, roast beef, veggies and salad, cake, wine and coffee at will. It really is a very well organized event!

Peter bought a bottle of champagne and on the ring of midnight, we will pop the cork and toast to the New Year. Two minutes before midnight, I say to Peter:

"Sweetie, you have no idea how long I have been waiting for this ugly, ugly year of 2003 to end! I will take a handful of air and with all my strength, throw it as far as possible. In my mind, this handful of air represents 2003. I want to run away from this terrible year so fast; it has been one bad thing after the other. It is an obsession and I want to see it end once and for all! Can you understand Darling or do you think I am mad?"

"I understand very well my Love and believe me I do not for one second think that you are mad. I too will do the exact same thing! Together, we will through 2003 away with all our strength. Let us kiss and say 'adieu' to this horrible year! What do you think of that Sweetheart? "

"Oh Peter, it will be wonderful! Thank you sincerely for everything you do for me! I thank you for staying by my side throughout this ordeal, never complaining; even when we had to get up at 4H30 to be at the hospital. We have suffered so much! I love you Darling and I thank you for being YOU!"

Suddenly the DJ screams out in his microphone:
"Everybody, gather on the dance floor!
5; 4; 3; 2; 1; Happy New Year to all!"

At that instant, Peter and I take a 'handful of air' and throw it as far as we possible can. We wish one another 'Happy New Year 2004' and seal it all with a kiss.

We offer our best wishes to Andrée and Renald and exchange wishes with all our surrounding.

They all wish me health, health, health! It is delirious on the dance floor! It is total euphoria; it is the New Year's Eve party!

At midnight, they untie the nets that are hanging from the ceiling and let the balloons fly down. There are balloons all over the place! The paper ribbons tangle around the dancers, the flutes, the hats... What an atmosphere! Best of all, we are in 2004! What a delightful time we are having!

It is so good to see the people laughing, jumping of joy and screaming to be heard! I have the impression that, for a few seconds, the entire world smiles and is happy! At this exact moment, I feel revived!

When the noise calms down a bit, we return to our tables. I grab my cellular and try to find a quiet spot to call the children.

I call Lily who is celebrating New Year's Eve with her family. When she answers, I scream:

"My best wishes for a very Happy New Year to you and yours Darling! I hope you are all having a good time! Here at the dance Hall, it is total euphoria! I must say Lily that at this moment I really have the impression that the whole world is happy and smiling! I want to take this opportunity to thank you for everything you do for me. I love you Lily! You are super and I am very proud of you! Please let me talk with Marc-André and the children."

After having talked to everyone, I call Eric. There is so much noise, I have to scream: "I wish you a very Happy New Year Darling! If I go by the noise on the phone, I guess you are having quite a lively party yourself! Do you have the impression that at this precise moment, the entire world is smiling and happy? We can nearly touch the happiness around us! Thank you very much for all that you do for me. I love you Eric and I am very proud of you! Continue your celebration; we are doing the same here!"

I am so proud of my children; they are truly extraordinary!

When I return to the table, Andrée, Renald and Peter are waiting for me to pop the champagne.

Once our glasses are filled, the four of us rise and through the total euphoria, we toast to this New Year of 2004.

The festivities continue until the wee hours of the morning. What a night!

Christmas and New Year's Eves are amongst the rare occasions that keep us up until the wee hours of the morning. We are a lot more disciplined than that usually! Those two nights are very special!

It is as though each New Year Eve is better than the last. We had so much fun! One moment it is a rock 'n roll, the next a waltz followed by a mambo; we do not even have time to become tired. We simply want to have fun and a lot of it! On with the party!

Too soon, it is closing time! We all hug, say 'Good night' and go home. Once at home, I hardly have enough strength to take off my make-up and jump into bed to take a very well deserved rest...

What a relief for our poor feet after all the stepping-around they did all night!

It was a fantastic evening! What a great time we had! What a wonderful way to end the disastrous year that was 2003! Most and foremost, what ecstasy to be in 2004!

In my prayers this evening, I cannot help but think:
'Once again my Dear Lord, You have succeeded in making me laugh! For a few hours, You allowed me to forget all the pain that is eating me inside. You alone seem to be able to accomplish such exploits! Do I dare ask You to help me out of this terrible situation? Yes, tonight you give me this audacity! Please Dear Lord, help me!'

I fall into a deep sleep but tonight; no nightmares, only beautiful dreams filled with flutes, laughter and music.

This New Year Eve is very important and very special for me! I do not know if it is because we finally got ride of 2003! I do not know if it is because Peter and I are still together to salute 2004! I do not know if it is because I am still alive!

Let it be for one reason alone or for all of them reunited, to this date, the 2004 New Year Eve party is by far, the best and most marvelous I have ever lived. I can easily say that it is the climax!

We wake up at 10 o'clock! Our festive breakfast consists of bagels, cream cheese and smoked salmon. Of course, we must not forget our favorite champagne! What a delight!

The phone rings and again Lily offers us her best wishes for a very Happy New Year. She certainly wants to know all the details of last night's party.

The first thing I say:
"Oh Darling, what an evening, what a party; it was incredible! We came home at 4H30 this morning! Lily we had so much fun, it was unbelievable! Peter and I took a big handful of air and with all our strength; we threw it as far away as we possibly could. This was our way of getting rid of 2003! You have no idea how good it felt! Can you understand that Sweetheart?

198

No answer! I know very well that she understands and that she is crying. I hear Cassandra's little voice saying:
"Hello Mamie! I want to wish you both a very Happy New Year! Most of all, Mamie Darling, I wish you health, health and more health! I love you so much!"
"Thank you my little Treasure and a very Happy New Year to you too! Continue your hard work at school, Peter and I are so very proud of you Darling! We wish you health, happiness and success in you studies! I too love you very much!"

Karl-David comes on the line and offers us his best wishes.
"Thank you for your precious wishes! Peter and I also wish you a Happy New Year! Health, happiness and success in your studies! We are very proud of you! I love you Darling and I send you a big hug.

Karl-David passes the phone to his father who also wishes us the best for the New Year.

They all talk to Peter and offer him their best wishes. They take this opportunity to thank him for all he has done for me throughout this ordeal and express their great appreciation.

Peter is very touched and he thanks them for being there for me. He thanks them for giving me so much love, so much affection and most of all, for giving me so many reasons to continue fighting even more.

A few minutes later, Eric calls to reiterate his best wishes:

"Hello Mom! How are you feeling on this first New Year's morning? I wish you again a very Happy New Year filled with health, health and more health! You have been through so much and fought so hard! I love you Mom and I am proud of you!"

"I am very well, thank you; even though we did come home at 4H30 this morning! How nice of you to call back! I also wish you a very Happy New Year, health, happiness and success in your work. I love you Darling and again, thank you so much for everything that you do for me day after day."

He also talks to Peter and offers him his best wishes for this New Year. He thanks him for everything that he does for me and tells him how appreciative he is of his support and constant presence by my side.

Now it is René-Luc's turn to call and offer us his best wishes! He too is very happy that 2003 is finally in the past. He thanks Peter for taking such good care of me and adds:

"You know Peter, I do not know if I would have had the strength to go through all that you have lived these past three years. I thank you very much for all that you do for her!"

A few friends call! They all wish us the best and never forget to include; health, health and health! What a good feeling to receive all these good wishes! It touches me very much!

200

The rest of the day goes by quietly! At eight p.m., Peter cannot hang on any longer. His eyes keep closing and he falls asleep on his favorite chair. I am looking at television but, very fast, I too fall asleep!

I wonder why we are so tired! What reason could we possibly have...?

As time goes by, it is as though my negative thoughts are not as negative! I seem to find life a little more attractive and a little easier to handle.

Is it because it is the Holiday Season? Is it because of all these wonderful gatherings with our loved ones? Is it because God heard my prayer? It is impossible for me to say! Although I admit that, the knot that I had in my throat for so long is starting to diminish. I find I can breathe a little easier!

The following Sunday, Peter and I go dancing with Andrée and Renald. In the washroom, a woman comes towards me and says:
"It is so nice to see you dance together! You have so much grace, such complicity! You have something special and it is very inviting to look at you. You both seem so happy and so much in love! We cannot help but admire you! Please, tell me: what is your secret?"

I absolutely do not know this woman and I wonder what prompts her to speak to me this way! What can I answer but:
"Thank you! It is very kind of you!"

Of course, I am flattered but I am mostly stunned!

When I return to the table, I tell Peter what happened in the washroom.

He looks at me and says:

"Ah, but this is not the first time that it has happened! I also have received compliments like this before and like you, I thank them and I too am very flattered."

We both stay very 'humble'! But one must admit that it is very flattering to be addressed with such wonderful compliments...

For the year 2004, Peter and I have taken new resolutions! The first one is to go out and walk every day! Even to go and walk in shopping centers if it is too cold or slippery outside. The second resolution is to go dancing at least once a week if possible.

After having applied these great resolutions for approximately one week, one morning I get up with a soar throat. The following morning, it is Peter's turn to have a soar throat.

I guess that 'morally' it is very easy to take resolutions, but 'physically'; it does not seem to be that easy! Unfortunately, we must face the fact; we are not that young anymore! What a pity!

Peter's cold gets so bad that we decide to go and see his Doctor. She sends him for a lung x ray and asks him to bring the x ray back to her office.

After examining the x ray, she says:
"You have a bronchitis accompanied with a sinus infection; I will prescribe antibiotics! You should drink a lot of liquids and most of all, get plenty of rest."

Well, this means 'goodbye' to our good resolutions, for this year anyway!

That same evening, René-Luc calls and asks how we are. I tell him:
"We were at the Doctor's today and Peter has a bad bronchitis and a sinus infection. She prescribed antibiotics and gave him a few days of complete rest. He honestly does not feel well at all and I am worried."

"I am sorry to hear that, but do not worry too much, he is very strong! I am calling because I am organizing a family reunion with all my sisters and brothers (he has 11 sisters and brothers) for the end of this month. I thought it would be nice if both of you could attend."

I am surprised and I wonder why he is inviting us. I say:
"René-Luc, do you realize that I have not seen your sisters and brothers for many years. Actually, it has been sixteen years! I do not understand your invitation!"

"When I called everyone, they all asked if you would be there! I told them I was hoping that you would! They are anxious to see you and to meet Peter. They always ask how you are and the children and I keep them informed! Will you come?"

"Honestly René-Luc, I would very much like to see them again, but do you not think that Peter and I would be misplaced? We have been separated for so long! I do not think that we would fit in! It is very nice of you to think of inviting us and we are both thankful; but I would not feel very comfortable. You do understand?"

"For the family, you will always be the Mother of Lily and Eric! They have always considered you as a member of the family. They would really like to see you. What do you say?"

"I cannot promise anything! I have to wait and see how Peter will feel in a few weeks. We will let you know!"

"I simply want to add that Lily and Eric would be very happy if you would come! They have already told me so!"

It goes without saying that Peter and I did not go out for several days! We stayed quietly at home in the heat!

One night, Eric comes over after work and invites us for supper. Peter is still not very well and prefers to stay home. He says:

"Listen Cookie, I really do not feel strong enough to go out. You should go with Eric! A little outing will do you a lot of good!"

Before I leave, I make sure that Peter has everything he needs and off we go.

We talk of different things and inevitably, the conversation comes to the family dinner that René-Luc is organizing.

"You know Mom, it will be a very nice gathering and Lily and I would really like it if both of you were there. Notwithstanding the fact that the entire family would like to see you again after all that has happened. What do you say Mom, will you come?"

"Darling, I told your Father I would think about it. Besides, I want to see how Peter will feel. You now Sweetheart, he is really in bad shape right now!"

When we come home, Peter is sleeping like a baby! Eric and I sit in the living room and he keeps me company for a while. I find this so wonderful to be able to talk of everything with the children!

In mid-January, I meet the Oncologist. After his meticulous examination, he looks at me and says:

"I am very satisfied with the exam! To date, all seems normal and your blood tests are normal. For the time being, you seem to have a nice quality of life and as long as it goes on this way, continue as you do. If something occurs, we will deal with it then! At the beginning of March, I would like you to undergo a stomach ultrasound; simply as a follow-up to the December exam. In the meantime, if anything worries you, please do not hesitate to call us immediately."

Peter and I come out of his office happy and satisfied with the visit! We decide to continue having as much fun as possible!

I call the children to give them the results of the visit! They are both happy to see that all is good, at least for now. We have to say that deep down inside we cannot help thinking of the disastrous December visit. We always have this fear that haunts us constantly and we cannot help ourselves thinking:
"When will this awful sickness come back?"

We often relive that drastic moment when the Doctor told us that the cancer was incurable. It is very oppressing to live with this constant thought on our minds!

We want to make our lives as full and happy as possible and take advantage of our loved ones. We try to be together often and do our best to keep positive thoughts.

In spite of all our efforts, this fear is anchored in every one of us. We simply cannot chase it away!

I knit, I sew, I play on the computer, I crochet, I really do my best to keep busy at all times hoping that it will deliver my mind from this sickness that tortures me so!

To top it all, Peter is not getting any better! I feel so depressed! I think my nerves are leaving me and that my determination to fight is weakening by the minute.

We went through so much and fought so hard, how can we let go now? Not after all the suffering! How can I avoid falling into a depression? I cannot find the strength to hold on! I feel caught in a stranglehold!

I do not want to disappoint everyone, not now! I have to regain control of my head and of my mind. I cannot stay like this! I must do something!

What can I do? I do not even know where to begin! There is only darkness in my head. Everything is so negative! I cannot pull myself together! There must be a way! I absolutely have to find a way!

A few days go by, yet nothing changes! I still do not feel good inside. The children notice the change; they can feel it in my voice. They keep asking:
"What is wrong Mom? Has something happened that you have not told us? Did you find another lump? What is bothering you? What is on your mind Mom? We feel it in every word you say! Please tell us!"

I keep repeating that everything is fine, that there is no new lump. I try very hard to change the subject, but it is useless.

I also can feel in their voices that they are very worried. I honestly do not know what to tell them to ease their worry. I hurt so bad inside yet I cannot find the words to explain this pain.

The following Saturday, Peter seems to feel a little better. I suppose that the antibiotics have started to work.

The telephone rings and Peter answers. He turns towards me and says:
"It is Lily and Eric, they are downstairs!"

As soon as they enter the room, I can feel how tense they are. It hurts me terribly to see them suffer this way! They look at me and wait until I say something. I cannot find the words! I really want to reassure them! I cannot come out saying that I think I am having a nervous breakdown! I am so confused and mixed-up; I do not know where to start.

How can I put in words what I feel inside? How can I make them understand that fear is eating me up? What comforting words can I find to ease their pain? I am unable to talk! They sit in front of me without saying a word; they just stare! I can almost see everything that is going on in their heads! With a tremendous effort, finally I say:

"Seriously Children, there is nothing wrong, at least nothing physical, honestly! As I told you this morning, the Doctor was very happy with the results of my tests and the exam on the last visit. All this is in my head! I am anguished and very nervous! We all are. I seem to suffocate and choke inside! I cannot stop thinking that the cancer could recur at any time. It must be because of the bad news we received last December when the Doctor told us I was incurable. So please, stop worrying over this. I am going through a bad period right now. I have to give it time, it will pass; I assure you it will. Now that Peter is feeling a little better, I am sure that in a few days things will be better. Please, stop worrying!

They both look at me very quietly; it is as though they are trying to analyze every word I said. Lily says:

"Mom, it is extremely difficult for all of us to live with such bad news! We are all very worried and very scared. Mom, you cannot give up now, you have always been so strong! You fought so hard, you cannot let go Mom, not now! Why not try to go out more often? It might be a good distraction and would do you both a great deal of good. What do you say? Will you at least try? You might say that it is easy for me to talk like this and I understand. Mom, you have to do something; you cannot stay in this state of mind!"

"I know Darling and I assure you that I do my utmost best to keep busy and distract myself as much as I can. I try to do all kind of things! Although, I think that you may be right in saying that we should try to go out more often. I promise that Peter and I will work very hard to recover a good moral and keep positive thoughts. So please, I beg of you, stop worrying, agreed?"

During the following week, Eric comes by a few times and Rick comes for a nice long visit with us.

I wonder if Peter or maybe Lily or Eric informed Rick of what was going on! Whatever, it is nice to have him with us for a few hours and it is very good for Peter. We had a wonderful time with him!

Now, it is Lily's turn to invite us to have lunch with her. On the way back home, Peter and I stop at the shopping centre and he buys me a beautiful pair of leather pants. They are really nice and they fit like a glove. I have wanted leather pants for such a long time and I am very happy.

They really do their utmost best to help me get out of this negative impasse! Their efforts are rewarded because towards the end of the week I feel a little better.

Finally, Saturday January 21st is here; it is the family reunion organized by René-Luc. I honestly have no desire to go and I cannot stop thinking:

'It has been over sixteen years that I have not seen them! I know that emotionally it will be very hard and I wonder if I am strong enough to survive such emotions, especially at this time. I honestly do not know what to do!'

I discuss it with Peter and he says:

"Listen Cookie; why not go to this diner? I am sure that they will all be very happy to see you. You told me that you know them since your childhood, that you even babysat their children when you were younger. How can they not be happy to see you after so many years, even more so after all that has happened these past three years? Once we get there and if you feel uncomfortable, we will simply come home. It is not more complicated than that! What do you say, do you want to try?"

"We will go; but if I find it too difficult, we will come home, you promise?"

"Yes Darling, I promise!"

When we arrive at René-Luc's place, everyone is already there and they greet me like a queen! It feels good and it is as though we saw one another last night. Conversation is easy and it is so nice to see them all again.

René-Luc offers a glass of champagne and we toast to this grand reunion! We serve ourselves to the nice buffet/diner that he has prepared. It is simply delicious! Eric plays the role of Maitre D and I have to admit that he is doing a great job!

The evening goes by very fast! I am happy that Peter convinced me to come to this magnificent family gathering.

In order to continue our good resolution of going out more, Peter and I decide to go dancing the following Saturday night. Andrée and Renald are there and, once again, we have a wonderful evening.

The children might be right when they say that distraction is the key to cure depression!

XIII

The relapse...

One week later, on Sunday morning while I am taking a shower and as I wash my neck, suddenly I feel a little lump on the left side. The lump is very tiny, really no bigger than a pea but when I touch it, it is very hard and also very painful.

There we go! The truce is over!

Now I know why I was feeling so anguished and depressed; the whole thing was in preparation! Peter could not understand my ups and downs and as previously, neither could I. When we think about it, to this day, this has always been the way it starts.

At the very beginning when I had all the exams, my attitude had changed tremendously. This time again, I had this fear that was destroying me and I was sliding more and more into a depression. Now we all understand; a new lump has made its appearance!

212

I do not tell anyone yet; I prefer to wait a while! I pray God that this is a mistake; that it is simply an illusion, not really a lump...

I verify my neck over and over! I pray for a miracle to happen; that the lump will disappear. Unfortunately, the lump is always there and it even grew after a few hours.

I am anxious for tomorrow morning to call my guardian Angel. I must inform her of what is happening in order for her to tell the Oncologist about it.

That night I am unable to sleep! It is like a video turning and turning in my head. Will it never stop?

I constantly think about this lump and I am so afraid that it is a relapse of the sickness! Incapable of sleeping, I get up and sit by the phone. I am desperately waiting for eight o'clock to call my guardian Angel.

Finally, eight o'clock and I dial! When she answers, she recognizes my voice and says:
"Good morning, you are very early this morning, is there anything wrong?"
"Good morning! Saturday night we went dancing! I had taken a shower, made-up my face and everything was fine. Yesterday morning, I took a shower and while washing my neck, I felt something on the left side. The lump is no bigger than a small pea and very hard. I feel my neck constantly praying for a miracle but it is not a dream, the lump has doubled. I am panicking!"

She understands and knows very well that if I call this early in the morning, there has to be something terribly wrong. She says:
"I will call the Oncologist immediately and explain the situation. As soon as I reach him and he tells me what he decides to do in this case, I will call you right back."

Fifteen minutes pass by, then half an hour; still nothing! I walk up and down in the living room.

When Peter gets up, I start giving him the details of what is going on. Needless to say that he too is very nervous! We wait impatiently for the phone to ring.

Forty minutes later, my guardian Angel calls back and says:
"The Doctor wants to see you after tomorrow at eight o'clock. He wants to verify the lump himself as soon as possible."

Wednesday morning Peter and I arrive at the hospital at 6H45 a.m. Because of the heavy traffic, we have to leave earlier to make sure that I will be on time for my eight o'clock appointment. I am so stressed and so worried; it is incredible! The lump keeps growing and growing. It has tripled since Sunday morning! I know my cancer is very aggressive but I never thought it would grow this fast.

Once in the Doctor's office, he examines my neck immediately. He is stunned to see how big the lump is and how fast it grew! He looks at my guardian Angel and says:

"Could you please schedule appointments with the O.R.L. Ward and also tests for a Gallium scan, an electrocardiogram, an abdominal ultrasound and a lung x ray? All these tests must be made today and tomorrow! I want her to start a treatment of 'Rituxan' (a kind of chemotherapy but not as violent and less harmful) as soon as Friday morning. With the aggressiveness of her cancer, we do not have one minute to lose!"

Looking at me, he says:
"I will prescribe anti-inflammatory pills to help reduce the inflammation and the swelling of the lump in your neck. You should be able to pass several tests today and most probably the rest of the exams could be done tomorrow. I really want you to get the first treatment of 'Rituxan' on Friday."

My guardian Angel is already on the phone making the appointments. Peter and I go to the Radiology Ward for the lung x ray and she meets us there. She gives me all the hours of my tests and the hour of my first 'Rituxan' treatment.

I pass two more tests that afternoon. My lymphoma is very aggressive and must be treated immediately. As the Doctor said, I really do not have one minute to lose.

Peter and I finally arrive home a little after seven p.m.; we are both bushed! Poor Sweetie, he followed me all day from one Ward to the other! What a day!

The following morning, we are back to the hospital for eight o'clock! I had to fast since midnight last night.

After the abdominal ultrasound, that finished at 3H15 p.m., they finally allow me to have a pop soda. What luxury! I still have one more exam before we can go home. Another very long and strenuous day!

Once we get home, Peter heats my 'miracle soup' and it is delicious! We are both exhausted and stressed and we try to relax and play on the computer for a while. We really try to keep ourselves as busy as possible. Even to play on the PC helps!

Everything and anything, as long as it distracts us enough and prevents us from constantly thinking of this disastrous sickness.

Two days in a row running around the hospital is very tiring and tonight again, we have to go to bed early. There is another full day waiting for us tomorrow and we must be well rested to face it!

Friday morning we arrive at the hospital at seven o'clock. We go to the Oncology ward and wait for the nurse to call me.

At 7H45 a.m., I hear my name on the microphone and go to Hall B for my treatment. While one nurse installs the serum, another one explains what will take place with the 'Rituxan'. She talks about the different side effects and their implications. After listening very carefully, I ask her:

216

"Will I lose my hair with this chemotherapy treatment? As of now, I have already lost them twice and I must say that I really did not enjoy the experience."

With a smile, she says:

"No, this time you should not lose your hair! This treatment should not make you sick either. You will become very tired and will probably lose your appetite. You will have to force yourself to eat at least one substantial meal a day. For the first two treatments, we will take you blood pressure every 15 minutes to make sure that all goes well. Do you have more questions?"

"Is it possible to give me an idea of the time it will take for the treatment, I have a meeting with the O.R.L. in the early afternoon."

"The first treatment is always a little longer! It lasts approximately 5H30 hours. The following treatments will last around 4H30 hours. But do not worry about your other appointment, if the treatment is not finished on time, we will call the O.R.L. and advise them of the delay."

I thank her.

Once they install the 'Rituxan' and after the nurse took my blood pressure several times, I look at Peter, who is always standing by my side, and say:

"Sweetie, I am all hooked-up and they are taking very good care of me. You should go to the cafeteria to eat something. You did not even have coffee this morning."

"I really prefer to stay here with you a little while longer. Besides I am really not hungry right now!"

For 5H40 p.m., I am hooked to a pouch of chemotherapy attached on a metal rod on wheels and I must drag my rod every time I need to go to the washroom. With the quantity of liquid they inject me; I must drag the rod very often. Overall, the first treatment goes quite well!

At 13H45 p.m., Peter and I go to the O.R.L. to meet with the Surgeon who will perform the biopsy. He examines me and says: "I will take a piece of the lump and have it analyzed. The results should give us a better idea of what is going on. I will perform the biopsy in eleven days. In the meantime, the hospital will call you to give you all the details. This is a one-day-in-hospital operation. I will see you the morning of the operation."

After the visit with the Surgeon, we have to go to the Cardiology Ward where I have to pass an electrocardiogram. Finally, after all this, we can go home.

I am very tired and once I get home, I go directly to bed. Peter wakes me up at around eight p.m. and serves me a nice hot bowl of my 'miracle soup'. I am really not hungry but I try to eat a little bit. Unfortunately, it simply will not go down! I go back to bed and Peter is discouraged. I feel very bad to see him like this, so I tell him:

"I am sorry Darling; but I am really not hungry! Please forgive me! "

He tucks me in and I fall asleep immediately. I spend the entire day of Saturday in bed and again today, Peter did not succeed in making me eat my soup.

In the evening, Lily calls and asks if she could come for a visit with the children and Marc-André the following day. Peter answers and tells her:

"Why not come over for pancakes tomorrow morning? It would be very good for your Mother and encourage her to eat a little bit. Besides, I know that it would please her very much to see all of you."

Sunday morning, Lily, Marc-André and the 'Mine-Mines, arrive at around 11 o'clock. We hardly have time to sit and start chatting that the phone rings and it is Eric who says he is downstairs. Approximately five minutes later, René-Luc knocks on the door. He offers me eighteen magnificent pink roses. I am very touched by his delicate attention! We all gather around the table and eat our favorite pancakes. Delicious!

They all leave at three o'clock and I go straight to bed. I am tired but very happy that they came! This helped me a lot and I even ate a little bit to the great pleasure of Peter.

I get up at around seven p.m. and Peter and I have a bowl of soup after which I go right back to bed. Thank God, at least I can sleep!

The following Tuesday, I have another appointment with the Oncologist. He is pleasantly surprised to see how fast the lump has diminished in such a short time. He agrees to the biopsy and asks to see me one week after the operation. He even qualifies me as a real 'box of surprises'...

I have another 'Rituxan' treatment scheduled on the eve of Valentine's Day. Peter and I buy a few boxes of chocolates for the personnel of the hospital.

We arrive at the hospital at 6H30 a.m. and go straight to the cafeteria. This time, Peter makes sure he has a good solid breakfast before heading for the Oncology Ward. He knows very well that he has four long hours of waiting ahead of him!

On our way out, we see a big bunch of Valentine's Day balloons and I buy five. When we get to the Oncology Ward, I give a box of chocolates to each secretary. They have always been so nice and kind to me. I also hang a balloon on each of their chair. After which I go looking for my guardian Angel and give her a box of chocolates.

They all have great smiles and thank me warmly for this delicate attention. This makes me feel very good!

As I enter the chemotherapy room, I hang the three balloons I have left to the nurse's desk. Three little balloons, it is not much and yet it creates such a joyful ambiance!

Even the patients that enter the Ward have a nice smile on their faces when they see the balloons. Five little balloons that create such great smiles and so much happiness! What a wonderful reward!

The nurse installs me for my treatment and 4H15 minutes later, Peter and I go the Nuclear Ward where I have to undergo an ultrasound. This test lasts over two hours and it is very strenuous. After all is done, we finally go home!

On Valentine's Day I get up at nine o'clock and Peter prepares a great breakfast. I still do not eat much but it is delicious and Peter is happy.

A little later in the day, Andrée and Renald call and ask Peter if we want to go dancing with them tonight. Peter answers that he will ask me when I wake up and we will call them back. When I get up, Peter says:
"Cookie, Andrée and Renald called and asked if we would like to go dancing with them tonight. How do you feel Sweetie? Do you feel strong enough to go out?"
"Why not Darling, we can at least try! If I get too tired, we will simply come home. Is that all right with you?"

I know that it will make him very happy! I call Andrée and say:
"Hello Andrée, how are you? How is Renald? Peter told me that you called and asked if we would like to go dancing with you tonight.

Listen, we will go but I honestly do not know how long we will be able to stay. I get tired quickly since I have the 'Rituxan' treatments, but I know that this will make Peter very happy. So, see you both later!"

Slowly, I start getting ready! Once ready, off we go for a fun evening.

Valentine's Day is always very special at 'Le Rendez-vous'! They serve a delicious meal and the dance Hall is all decorated in red and white. Needless to say that the place is completely full! They have white and red balloons all over the place and the atmosphere is electrifying.

Of course, Peter and I cannot dance very much, but simply being out with friends in such a wonderful ambiance, helps us a great deal. Around nine p.m. I get very tired and we have to go home.

Even if we came in early, Peter is very happy and this is what matters the most. It was really worth it and we had a real good time!

XIV

The biopsy...

The morning of the biopsy, Peter and I arrive at the hospital for six o'clock and as requested by the surgeon, I was not allowed to eat nor drink since midnight. We go to the 6th floor and inquire at the nurse's desk. One nurse takes me to a room and tells me to put on the hospital gown.

She tells me:

"I will be back in a little while to take your blood pressure and blood tests.

As soon as I am ready Peter joins me and we chat while waiting for the nurse.

An hour and a half later, the nurse enters the room and says:

"The surgeon received several emergencies this morning that he needed to deal with; therefore your operation has been delayed. As soon as they call us, we will take you down."

She takes my blood pressure and blood tests and adds:

"The Cardiology technician will come by for an electrocardiogram."

Finally they take me down to the operating room at 1H30 p.m. Because Peter cannot come with me, he goes to the cafeteria. I have total anesthesia for this operation and return to my room at 5H30 p.m.

Poor Peter he spent all afternoon on a chair waiting for me! I had suggested that he go home and return towards the end of the afternoon, but he refused. He said:
"No Darling, I really prefer to stay here and wait. I want to be in the room when you return from the operation."

The nurse takes several blood tests and takes my blood pressure every fifteen minutes. I have a huge dressing around my neck and the nurse also says that I have a tube to drain the puss.

I ask her:
"When can we go home? We are both so tired and we simply want to get out of here and go home."
"You are still too weak and your blood pressure is way too low. We cannot let you go in those conditions. We must wait for your blood pressure to stabilize and for you to gather more strength. Be patient Madame and try to rest; it would help stabilize your blood pressure. Besides, you need to see the surgeon before we can let you go! He is the only one who can sign your release."

I can see that Peter is also tired and anxious to get back home to rest. What can I do? I must wait!

At eight o'clock p.m., the surgeon finally comes through the door and asks how I am feeling. I know I am still very weak but I so much want to go home. He says:
"Once your blood pressure is stabilized, I will allow you to go home. I cannot sign your release before! I want to see you tomorrow morning at seven o'clock to change your dressing and remove the drain if necessary."

Finally, they release me at 9H30 that evening! Peter takes me to the car in a wheelchair. Once in the garage, I am so weak that I can hardly make it to the apartment. Peter has to help me to the bed, covers me and I am fast asleep!

The following morning, we are back to the hospital at 6H30 a.m. To our amazement, the Doctor is leaning on the reception desk and he is waiting for me. He takes me to a little room, removes the dressing, verifies the drain and makes another dressing; quite smaller this time. While doing so he says:
"I will remove the dressing and the drain on your next visit. Should the wound start bleeding, you must come to the Emergency Ward immediately!"

At 8H30 in the morning, we are en route for home! What a change when we compare to the other late nights!

I spend all day in bed! I feel very bad! Peter heats up some of my 'miracle soup' for lunch and diner; the soup is the only thing I seem to be able to swallow.

As the dietitian was saying:
"Thank God it is very nutritious!"

Since the biopsy, the children call us every day. They are worried and want to know how Peter and I are doing. They always ask if they can do anything for us.

The day after the biopsy Eric comes over for a visit, but seeing that I am sleeping, he chats with Peter for a while and leaves.

The children ask if they could come for a visit on Saturday. I am sure that by then I will feel a little better!

Three days after the operation, Peter and I are back to the hospital for my third treatment of 'Rituxan'.

Everything goes quite well and around noon, we are on our way back home. We rest all afternoon and believe me; we both needed that time-off!

All these daily visits to the hospital are extremely tiring; notwithstanding the wait, the stress and the anguish... Needless to say, that we are both exhausted!

On Saturday morning, Lily, Marc-André and the 'Mine-Mines' arrive at ten o'clock and offer me a beautiful arrangement of flowers. Not even half an hour later, Eric knocks on the door and offers me a big bouquet of flowers!

When Peter goes to the kitchen to prepare lunch, Eric joins him and they cook up a delicious meal. It is so nice to see them work side by side! This is a very good visit and we both appreciate it very much.

They all leave at three o'clock and the doorbell rings at 3H 30. It is René-Luc and he too offers me a dozen beautiful yellow roses. They spoil me too much; but believe me: I am not complaining; I take it all in!

They are all so kind! They really try their utmost best to make life as beautiful as possible. Peter and I greatly appreciate their efforts and their numerous attentions! What a formidable team we have surrounding us! Dear God we are blessed to have such good people encourage and support us!

When Rick calls, Peter gives him the latest news. Rick has been traveling a lot these past few weeks; right now, he is calling from New Jersey. He promises Peter he will come by as soon as he gets back in town. Peter needs and enjoys his visits so much! What a super day; it was awesome!

All these delicate attentions are very stimulating and they give me even more reasons and strength to continue my battle against this deadly disease.

Whether the days are good or bad, we never forget to thank God for all He does. Somewhere He gives us a reason to smile and allows us to live great fulfilling moments!

Sunday afternoon Andrée and Renald come by and bring me a big bouquet of flowers. The living room is filled with gorgeous flowers! What wonderful aroma they spread in the room.

They are not very long because they do not want to tire me! It was very nice of them to drop by and we enjoyed their visit very much. We really appreciate their precious friendship!

The rest of the day is quiet and I even play a little on the computer. Peter heats up some soup for diner and as soon as I finish eating, I go to bed.

My guardian Angel calls Monday morning and says:

"The appointment that was scheduled with the Oncologist for tomorrow has been postponed for two weeks. The Doctor is out of town for a conference and has decided to take an extra week for vacation. In the meantime, should anything occur, please do not hesitate to call me and I will make arrangements for you to see another Oncologist."

What can I say? Of course I much rather see my own Oncologist for the follow-ups! But if something does happen, I will not hesitate to see another Doctor. For the time being, everything seems to be under control!

As for the biopsy, the operation was a total success. I can surely wait until the Oncologist returns! Besides, this will give us both a well-deserved rest from the hospital!

On Tuesday morning, Lily calls and asks: "Mom, do you feel strong enough to come over for diner tonight?"

I discuss it with Peter and he agrees!

Before going to Lily's we stop to pick-up Cassandra at the bus stop then we go and get Karl-David in his schoolyard. When we arrive at Lily's, Marc-André is already home. While Peter chats with Marc-André, I am in the living room chatting away with the 'Mine-Mines'.

I enjoy talking with them so much! They are really interesting! Unfortunately, I find that they are growing up way too fast! Cassandra is already a young woman and Karl-David a wonderful young man.

Lily comes in from work and she is happy to find us there. We chat while the children set the table and in no time at all, diner is served. How nice it is to be all together like this!

During the meal, I ask Lily:
"Darling, would you agree to let us have the children for a few days during their spring break?"
"Mom, are you sure that you are strong enough?"
"Of course Darling, they are both grown-up now and furthermore, Peter is there. Do not worry, everything will be fine! Should something happen, you know that I will call you right away."

We leave for home at around 8H30 p.m., both happy and satisfied.

Friday morning we are both at the hospital for eight o'clock for my fourth 'Rituxan' treatment. Once again, everything goes fairly well!

After the treatment, we meet with the Surgeon to change, or I hope, to remove the dressing and the drain. He removes the dressing and the drain and he covers the wound with surgical plasters. He says:
"As soon as the results of the biopsy come in, I will send them to the Oncologist."

The following Monday morning, Lily brings the children to stay with us for a few days. We all eat together and a couple of hours later, Lily goes home.

The children stay with us until Wednesday. We have so much fun with them and enjoy the delicious meals that Peter prepares for us. The children never complain about Peter's cooking; to the contrary, they qualify him as an 'excellent cook'.

Wednesday at lunchtime, Peter and I decide to take the kids to the restaurant for lunch before driving them home. They like going to restaurants and it is very normal at their age.

While the children were staying here with us, Lily decided to paint her living room and dining room.

When we enter the apartment, we all have a shock! We have the impression that we are in the wrong apartment!

I really wonder where she takes the strength and the courage to paint at night after a full day's work. God knows her days at the office are awfully busy! She says that not only does she love to paint but also that it relaxes her. To say the truth, I know no one who finds that painting is relaxing...

On Sunday morning the phone rings and it is Andrée. She is all excited. I ask her:
"What is going on Andrée? Did you win the lottery?"
"I have such great news to tell you! I am sure that you will never guess!"
"What on earth can it be?"
"Renald and I are getting married! We will celebrate our engagement on Easter and marry on my 60th birthday; October 9th. What do you say about that?"
"Congratulations! I am so happy for both of you. Tell me, when was all this decided?"
"We had talked about it a few times! One morning while we were at our favorite restaurant, one of the waitresses was making jokes to the effect of:
'... to have children, you must be married...'
So I look at Renald and jokingly I say:
'Well my Love, we will simply have to get married!'
Very seriously, he replies:
'Give me at least one week to think about it! Marriage is a very serious matter you know!'
The following week he tells me:

231

'After giving it a serious thought, I agree; let's get married!'
If only you knew how happy I am, you have no idea! We wanted you to be the first two people to learn about it."
"Dear Andrée, this is really fantastic news! Let us be the first to offer our most sincere congratulations. We are so happy for you!"

Peter and I are very happy for them! They started dating about four and a half years ago, and as I know Andrée for more than fifteen years, I can understand her happiness now. What marvelous news!

Even though we are going through a very difficult period at this moment, one way or another, there is always something that happens that warms our hearts and makes us smile. When we think of it, life is awesome! It is really worth living and fighting for; even with its ups and numerous downs...

The following Tuesday, I meet with the Oncology specialist for the results of the biopsy. He will also give me the results of all the other tests I have passed. Once we are sitting in his office, he says:
"The Surgeon who made your biopsy said that the piece of lump that he removed for analysis, has returned negative; in other words, no lymphoma! On the other hand, the Gallium scan shows that the cancer is spreading. There is more sickness in your right hip and new sickness on both sides of your ribs."

Peter and I look at one another; we are totally stunned! Once again, we do not want to believe it! I look at the Doctor and like a robot, I scream:

"Oh my God, more bad news, will it always be like this? Will we always be hit with bad news? Will it never end? This is incredible; I have no idea of how much more I can take of such terrible and awful news. Now tell me Doctor, does this mean that the cancer is generalizing? Is this what you are trying to make us understand?"

"Yes, unfortunately this is exactly what it means; the cancer is generalizing! Right now, we are hoping that the 'Rituxan' treatments that you are receiving will help reduce the rapidity of the progression. They will help, that is for sure!"

"If I understand correctly; we are right back to February 2003, before the auto graft of the bone marrow. At that precise moment, you told us that as soon as I would get a lump; you would give me a treatment and so on and so forth... until there were no more treatments to be had! You also told us that my life expectancy would be between 18 to 24 months. Is this what we are coming back to today?"

"Dear Madame, I can understand that it is very difficult to receive such atrocious news! I promise that we will do our utmost best to help you and yours. We will try to make you as comfortable as we possibly can."

Suddenly an idea crosses my mind like the flash of lightening. Peter and I had talked about this a few times before: go on a trip to Paris...

I have already been to Paris several times before. For a reason completely unknown to me, I have the strong feeling that seeing Paris with Peter would be very different. I cannot explain why I feel so strongly about this, but this is the way I feel.

Following my idea, that is becoming clearer in my mind and without hesitation, I look at the Doctor and say:
"Doctor, do you think we still have time to make plans?"

He stares at me and this time he is the one that is stunned! He really does not know where on earth I am going with such a question especially after having given us such terrible news. He asks:
"What plan are you talking about?"
"Go on a trip!"
"Go on a trip? Where do you want to go?"
"We would like to go to Paris!"
"Paris! Are you serious? How long would this trip be?"
"If at all possible, we would like to go for approximately one month, but it goes without saying that I need your approval."
"This is indeed a very big project Madame! To tell you the truth, I absolutely cannot give you an answer right now. I must wait a while!

Firstly because we have to see what effect the 'Rituxan' treatments will have on you and secondly, we have to wait to see how you will feel in a few weeks. This is quite a big undertaking! I am not saying 'NO' but I really cannot say 'YES' either; at least not at this precise time. I hope you can understand!"

"Yes Doctor, I understand! Your answer is very clear and quite normal especially after giving us such bad news concerning the cancer. Thank you; at least you did not say 'NO'! I still can have hope!"

Peter and I leave his office! I am very much aware of the fact that we have received very negative news and yet, this is not what I am thinking about right now. I cannot help thinking that the Doctor did not say 'NO' to my project. He simply asked us to wait a little while longer! He wants to see how things will develop before deciding!

I honestly feel very excited inside! The positive 'probability' of this trip seems to take the upper hand on the 'official' negative of the bad news concerning the cancer. I have to admit that I really do not understand my reasoning and the way I feel right now and yet, this is the way it is.

Once at home, I am in no hurry to call the children. To have to give them more bad news; oh no, I am really in no hurry at all! I will call them, because I promised I would; but I need to wait a while and try to deal with this!

Peter and I talk about the visit we had with the Doctor and we try to cheer ourselves up with the trip to Paris. He cannot get over the fact that after receiving such horrific news; I can even think of such a preposterous idea and more so, that it can rejoice me so!

Several hours after our return, I think that it would be the right time to call Lily and Eric and give them the bad news!

I am so sad and unhappy to have to give them negative news once again! I wonder how they will react!

First, I call Lily and inform her of our visit with the Doctor this morning. Then I call Eric and give him the bad news. I cannot help asking myself how much more they can endure of all these ups and downs. I do not mention the trip to Paris because the answer is not official and besides, I know how much they suffer and how worried they are for me!

Once more, what can I do? It deeply hurts me to have to constantly give them bad news. I feel so helpless!

After talking with the children I feel I have to do something to distract myself otherwise I am going to go out of my mind. I sit at the computer and automatically go on Internet and start surfing for everything and anything I can find on Paris. Hotels, maps, cost of flights, places to visit; actually all I can find! This keeps me busy for several hours and believe it or not, it becomes an obsession.

The time I spend 'in Paris', on Internet, is very beneficial for me! It takes my mind away from all the negativity I find myself in right now. Lord knows I need a change! I do not want to succumb into another depression...

The following morning, we are back to the hospital to meet the Hepatitis specialist. I see him regularly since the auto graft of the bone marrow. As far as the Hepatitis is concerned, he is satisfied with the tests and the blood tests are good. He schedules another Rendez-vous and we leave.

Once at home, my guardian Angel calls saying:
"The Doctor has decided to stop the 'Rituxan' treatments. He thinks that four treatments should be enough for the time being. He wants to see what impact they will have."

Instead of going back to the hospital the following morning for the 'Rituxan' treatment, Peter and I decide to go for our passport photos and pick-up the forms at the same time. As soon as we return home, I fill-out the forms! I am happy and excited and yet, I do realize that this is probably just a dream. But it is MY dream and I will not let anyone take it away from me. It is mine and I am going to hang on to it with all the strength I have.

Right now, I need to cling to this dream more than anything else in the world. We all have a right to dream, even I; maybe more so than anyone else! I live in my dream!

Life can be very funny sometimes! Here the Doctor gives me the worst news of all and instead of being struck down with sadness and despair, as I should be with such devastating news, I tightly hang on to a 'maybe' and I live each hour in the only hope that my 'unrealistic' dream might come true!

Peter does not understand! Of course, he is ecstatic to see that I am not sinking into a huge depression... On the other hand, he cannot understand my reaction!

Eric comes over for diner on Saturday night and I tell him about my project, making sure to mention that the Doctor has not yet said 'YES'. I tell him that we simply want to be ready in case he does! Down deep inside, Eric knows very well that this is an impossible dream, but he says nothing. I guess he does not want to take away the only joy I have left. I show him the passport forms and he verifies them closely. He says that he will have one of his friends certify them for us.

After diner, we watch a hockey game! We have a wonderful time! Eric's presence fills the entire place and gives me great joy. It is incredible how good it feels to be surrounded by my loved ones!

Sunday, around lunchtime, Andrée calls and asks if we feel like going dancing tonight. As we are both very anxious to have more details on their up-coming wedding, we decide to meet them at the dance Hall.

As soon as we meet them at 'Le Rendez-vous', we can see the happiness in their faces! We are so interested in every detail of their wedding arrangements that we even forget to dance. It is awesome!

All of a sudden, the four of us turn towards the end of the table and see Eric standing there. I ask him:

"Darling, what are you doing here?"

"I am returning your passport forms! As promised, my friend certified them and they are ready. All you have to do now is take them to the Passport office."

I present Eric to Andrée and Renald and I thank him. We hug and he leaves!

Andrée and Renald stare at us with interrogations in their eyes. We relate our visit with the Oncologist this week and inform them of our project. They are overwhelmed and very excited for us.

Andrée says:

"I suppose that the simple fact of hoping for the possibility of realizing such a project must excite you both very much."

"It sure does! Since we have talked to the Doctor about this project and even though he has not yet agreed to it, I still have hope. Of course, there is always the terrible news that my cancer is generalizing that preoccupies us very much; but the possibility of making such a trip seems to overcome the terribly bad news. This dream fills me with joy!"

We have a wonderful time and the evening is full of great projects.

On Monday morning, we go the Passport office and give them the passport forms.

The woman at the counter says:
"Your passports will be returned to you via registered mail. You should receive them in approximately two weeks."

When we come out of the Passport office, we stop at the pastry store and order a birthday cake for Cassandra and Karl-David.

Lily and Marc-André have invited us for diner this coming Friday to celebrate their anniversaries. Their birth dates are very close even if there is a four-year-age difference.

Friday afternoon we pick-up the cake and go to Lily's. Eric and his girlfriend arrive a little while later and we have a wonderful time all together. The 'Mine-Mines' enjoy their party and their birthday presents.

We talk about our 'Paris' project. Everybody is very happy to see me so upbeat and content and cannot get over to see me so enthused. Eric says:
"Mom, even if the Doctor has not yet said 'YES' to the trip, at least the time that you spend on the computer making all your researches keeps you from constantly thinking about your sickness. This can only be positive for you! We are all so happy that this dream occupies your mind so much! I can really feel it Mom, it fills you up with hope! It is fantastic!

240

This is already the third anniversary that we celebrate with my little 'Mine-Mines' since my death sentence in 2001. Sometimes, I can hardly believe that I am still alive and able to appreciate all these precious moments. I often have the impression that I am living on borrowed time and this gives me a very funny feeling; but I love it!

Whatever the length of my life may be; short or long, I want to bite into it and take total advantage of everything that goes on around me. I feel privileged to be part of this beautiful world! What a great gift God gives me day after day!

Sunday morning Lily calls all excited. She screams on the phone:

"Mom, you will never guess what my daughter and I did this morning! We had our belly buttons pierced. It was fantastic!"

"Ouch! That must have been very painful!"

But immediately I add:

"You must not pay any attention to me, I am an old Mamie and in my time, we would have never imagined doing such a thing! Well, if this made you both happy, why not?"

"Not only am I extremely happy to have done this with MY daughter but I am also very proud of it. Can you imagine Mom? I find this extraordinary!"

"I am really very happy for both of you especially if it pleased you so. On the other hand, be careful of the infection!"

Ever since I have been so sick, I have a real phobia about infections and because of this; I could not help myself but beg them to be very careful!

I continue browsing on the Internet. I make copies of several packages, I regroup different sectors of Paris and I tape them together and make a map. Peter cannot get over to see all the trouble I am giving myself, but I am having so much fun and it really gives me great pleasure to do all this! I know what you are thinking:

"Why give yourself so much trouble? You can easily buy a road map of all the streets in Paris anywhere!"

You are absolutely right! If only you knew the immense satisfaction this procures me, you would understand. I also take notes of the different places we might like to visit and of everything I find interesting. This occupies me day after day and it keeps my mind off the cancer that is growing inside me. Actually, all I want is to occupy my mind!

Eric comes by as often as he can and Lily calls every day for news.

René-Luc calls and says:

"I am having a brunch on Easter Sunday with the kids and I was wondering if you and Peter would accept to join us?"

"Thank you for thinking of us! You know that it is always a pleasure for Peter and I to attend your receptions but I cannot answer right now.

Our dear friends Andrée and Renald have invited us for their engagement party. I still do not have the exact date of the event. If it is not on Easter Sunday, of course we will join you! I will call Andrée and as soon as I have the exact date, I will call you back."

I call Andrée and say:

"Hello Andrée! How are you? Are you always happy? How is Renald? I am calling to ask if you have settled on your engagement date."

"We are both very well thank you! And 'yes' we are both always very happy! We wanted to celebrate the event on Easter Sunday but it was impossible to get a reservation at the restaurant we had chosen. Therefore, we decided to get engaged one week earlier. You are coming aren't you?"

"Of course we will be there! We promised, did we not? We would not miss this important event in the lives of our best friends. Be assured; we will be there!"

All is well that ends well!

I call René-Luc and gladly accept his invitation. The busier we will be, the better it will be for everyone...

The last Monday of the month of March, Peter and I go to the hospital to pass the lung x ray previously prescribed by the Oncology specialist.

Saturday, April 3rd, 2004, Andrée and Renald celebrate their engagement. We all agree to meet at the chosen restaurant!

Andree's sister and brother are there with their spouses. Renald's two daughters and his grandson are there. Renald's siblings are also there with their spouses plus a few friends of the couple.

We are all reunited around a table and with our spoons; we tap on our glasses at the request of kisses from the newly engaged couple as we do at weddings. We have so much fun!

The evening is a total success! The happiness we read on their faces is contagious! They both look wonderful!

XV

The doctor says 'yes'...

Finally, April 6th, 2004 has arrived! Today is my meeting with the Oncology specialist. As Peter and I enter his office, we find him and my guardian Angel both wearing a huge smile on their faces. The Doctor says:
"The lung x ray has returned normal! The left side of your neck, where you had the biopsy, is healing very nicely and your blood tests are normal. Now tell me, are you still thinking of your trip to Paris?"
"We have not stopped thinking about it since our last visit. It is constantly on our minds! Why are you asking me this question?"
Without even waiting for the Doctor's answer, Peter adds:
"Doctor, I can assure you that should something occur during the trip, anything at all, we would take the first plane back! I promised her children that I would bring their Mother back home safely, and I will!"

The Doctor looks at Peter and with a smile gently says:

"Sir, I have never doubted that! You have never missed one Rendez-vous since the beginning of her sickness and not one day of visit during her numerous hospitalizations. I also know of your obsession to keep her alive. It reassures me to know that you will be with her throughout this trip and I am convinced that, should anything happen, you surely would not hesitate to come back. You are well aware of the aggressiveness of her cancer and the danger she faces if she delays being treated. Therefore, I wish you both a very good trip. Take advantage of every second, you deserve it so much!"

As of this famous 'YES' I become more and more addicted to life! I want to live every single second to the fullest.

As soon as we come out of the hospital, I cannot wait to call the children to, finally, give them the 'super' good news. It is about time! What a relief for me to hear them burst out laughing rather than feel them crying in silence. I am so happy!

Dear God, how can I thank The, I have no more words. A simple 'Thank You' simply does not seem to be enough! How can I lose my faith after so much kindness!

I call everyone to give them the good news! I am so excited and overwhelmed and Peter is all smiles to see me this happy.

Once we arrive home, I 'jump' on the computer and this time, not simply for fun! I am not simply browsing anymore... I note all the tickets and hotel prices, car rentals, everything I can find. Peter goes out and because I am so preoccupied with Paris, I do not even notice his absence ...

When he returns, his arms are filled with bags. I look at him stunned and say:
"Where have you been? I had not noticed your absence! What do you have in the bags?"
"Darling, this is such wonderful news that it deserves to be celebrated! I will prepare a feast for us fit for a queen. Thanks to you and your 'peculiar' ideas we are looking forward to the trip of our dreams, I can even say the trip of our lifetime... For lunch, we will have a bowl of soup and tonight, we will have a feast. What do you say my Love?"

The afternoon flies by very fast! Peter is in the kitchen preparing our delicious meal and I am on the Internet, I should say in Paris...

Around seven o'clock, I start dressing the table by placing, in the centre, the beautiful bouquet of 12 red roses and then our place settings without forgetting the candles.

When diner is ready, Peter serves a tender filet mignon, jumbo shrimps and rice on the side. When he sits at the table, he admires the flowers, the beautiful place settings and the candles. Suddenly, he looks at the wine glasses, turns towards me and cries out:

"Oh no Darling, not simple wine glasses tonight! We are celebrating such a great occasion! Tonight we have champagne and we need our beautiful flutes! I only want the best for you my Love!"

No sooner said, he jumps up, grabs the wine glasses and returns with the flutes and the well chilled champagne bottle.

We both stand up and toast to all the marvelous moments that are offered to us on a silver platter. We also toast to the realization and the success of this wonderful trip. At this exact instant, we are both totally content and overwhelmed!

Easter Sunday is here and we are on our way to René-Luc's brunch. When we arrive Lily, Marc-André, the 'Mine-Mines' and Eric are already there.

René-Luc fills the flutes and we toast to good health and the wonderful trip to come. After which we all gather around the table and savor a perfectly delicious meal. What do you think the main subject of discussion is? Paris of course! I narrate all the searches I made on the Internet including all the pieces I glued together to make a map. They all laugh! Eric looks at me and says:

"Mom, I have a Travel agent who does all my trip bookings; I am sure that he would be pleased to help you with your reservations. If you are interested, I could schedule and appointment with him next week."

"Of course we are interested! You see, not only are we thinking of going to Paris; we want to go to Germany to see Peter's brother and his family; then to Hungary where Peter was born. We also want to stop in Vienna and go to 'Stadt Park' to admire the professional dancers of Viennese waltzes. They give such a wonderful show in the gardens of a Hotel, when the weather permits. After all that, we want to stop in Munich; this time I absolutely want to go and see Lucie and her family. I have not seen Lucie in fifteen years and Achim, her husband, in eighteen years."

"Well Mom, I guess you absolutely need the help of the Travel agent to organize such an itinerary. I was not aware that you wanted to go around the world... Tell me Mom, how long do you plan to be gone to accomplish such a merry-go-round?"

"We plan to be gone for approximately one month. Of course, the Doctor agreed!"

They are all very happy for us! Most of all, they enjoy seeing me laugh, happy and all excited. We spend such precious time together! Right now everything we do is good and marvelous.

Two days later, we meet the Travel agent and one and a half hour later, the whole trip is organized. He even reserved the shuttle that will take us from the airport to the Hotel. Peter and I are content with the arrangements and we are both satisfied!

It is really true! Everything is right there on paper! I can hardly believe it! I am floating; I am so happy! For Eric and Peter to see me jubilate like this brings tears to their eyes. They cannot believe that with all that is hanging over my head, I can be so vibrant and dazzling. Yet, I really am!

I keep thinking:

'I cannot let this sickness get the better of me and simply stop living! Besides, as long as my time is not up, I must continue to fight with all my might, have as much fun as I possibly can and be happy. May the Lord guide all our steps and give us strength!'

The following Saturday we meet our newly engaged friends at the dance Hall. We give them all the details of how fast the Travel agent organized our trip. We also give them all the details of the itinerary.

They are all ears and all smiles and are very happy for us! It is nice to have wonderful friends to share such happiness!

Rick comes over for pancakes on Sunday morning and we give him the details of our upcoming trip. He says:

"I am so happy for both of you! Take full advantage of each second and have a lot of fun! By the way, do you have an international cellular phone? It would be wise to have one! Once you come out of Paris, you will mainly be driving on autobahns; you might not find too many phone booths on the way!"

"That is a very good idea Rick, it never occurred to me! Thank you! Tomorrow morning I will call my cellular company and ask them what the possibilities are for them to arrange that for me. I hope they could come up with something! Thanks again and of course, we will see you before we leave!"

The following day; I call the cellular company and inquire on an international cellular phone. The woman says:
"The phone that you have now is not made for international calls. It is not strong enough to pick-up international waves. We will send you another cellular strong enough for the necessary waves and include the connections for the international networks. The package should arrive in about one week."

Slowly we start setting aside cloths and several articles that we absolutely want to take on the trip. I am still having a hard time believing that we will really realize this super big project.

I am constantly afraid that something might happen; something negative that would force us to change our plans or even worse; cancel the wonderful trip that we have been dreaming of for several months already. Dear God, please make sure that all goes well!

I try very hard to fight against this fright that is eating me up inside and I do my best to keep positive thoughts. But every day, it gets worse and worse!

I cannot sleep very well and even my appetite is affected! Poor Darling, he does his utmost best to calm me down! He tries so hard to help me control this fright that is within me. I keep telling him that it is very difficult to control fear and stress. He understands but nevertheless, he continues trying and does everything he can to keep me as occupied as possible hoping that I will think less. He follows me everywhere!

Lily calls and says:

"Mom, it is Karl-David's turn to have his First Communion and, as for Cassandra, I still do not have the exact date of the ceremony. As soon as they give us the date, I will let you know right away."

"Lily, I will pray very hard for the event to be before the 26th of April, date of our departure for Paris. I really do not want to miss this special event in my grandson's life. Peter and I really want to be there!"

I cannot help thinking:

'Life is funny sometimes! For Cassandra's First Communion I was afraid to be hospitalized and now for Karl-David's; I am afraid to be gone on a trip...'

A few days later, Lily calls back:

"Mom, finally I have the date! The First Communion is scheduled for Sunday April 25th. I know that you leave for Paris on the 26th, but do you think that you will be able to find time to come?"

"Oh Darling, you have no idea how relieved I am! I was so afraid that it might be at a later date. Honestly, I do not know what I would have done had it been the case. Sweetheart, you know very well that we would not miss this event for all the money in the world. Besides, we are only leaving on the 26th, we will have plenty of time to finalize the last-minute details and take the plane. Everything is perfect and do tell Karl-David that both Peter and I will be at the church on time."

Sunday April 25th and we are all gathered in the church for the event! This is a very special event for me and I am alive to appreciate it to the fullest. I am so grateful!

After the ceremony and several photos, we go to Lily and Mark-André's to celebrate. Lily ordered a beautiful buffet and we all enjoy ourselves. Everyone wishes us a very good trip and tell us to take full advantage of it. We promise the children to call them every week.

Around five o'clock, we kiss the children and the 'Mine-Mines' and head for home. We still have several last-minute things to put together before leaving tomorrow.

Once we get home, we finalize everything and buckle the suitcases. All of a sudden Peter takes my hand and says:
"Cookie, what would you say if we upgraded our tickets to first class?"
"Why are you asking me this now Darling? It is way too late!"

"First of all, because I know that you are very frightened of flying and second, have we not said that we wanted to make this trip the trip of our lives? This would be the perfect occasion, do you agree?"

"Sweetie, first class is very expensive and I doubt that at the last minute like this there would still be two first class tickets together. It is absolutely out of the question that I sit next to anyone else but you."

"I know very well that we must be seated together, but you could at least try to call the Travel agent and ask him if there are still first class tickets available and what would it cost? What do you say?"

Needless to say that neither Peter nor I were able to sleep last night! My head was spinning with all kinds of questions and it would not stop:

'Do we have everything we need for this trip? Are the passports, the plane tickets, the hotel reservations etc. in the right place? So many questions go through my mind! Will it ever stop spinning in there?'

Finally; the morning of the departure! Dear God, I thought it would never come! I have to say that it is not too soon because a few more days of this anxiety and I could have gone right back into another big depression!

We are on the 26th and to date, I am still in shape and I see no negative signs ahead! I really feel great!

Usually I check my neck, my throat and my head once or twice a day. Ever since the Doctor said 'YES' for this trip, it has been a lot worse. I constantly explore my head in search of... The closer we get to the departure date, the more I feel my head, the more I am frightened, the more I stress and the more I anguish.

Of course I am always very excited for the trip but until we are both sitting in the plane and well strapped in, I will not be able to stop touching my neck, my throat and my head in the case that I might find a 'lump'.

My dear Lord, I beg of You, please allow us to make this trip! Please guide our every step and protect us!

I wait until 9H30 a.m. to call the agent and say:

"Good morning Sir, would you kindly check to see if, by miracle, there are still first class tickets available and if so, would there be two seats together?"

"Miraculously, there are still two tickets left in first class and they are together! Seeing the imminent departure, it will only cost $100 more per ticket."

"Fantastic! Could you please make the necessary changes?"

"I already took care of it! All you have to do is present yourself to the first class desk for registration, everything is confirmed. Have a very good trip!"

Peter looks at me and says:
"Well Darling, all is well that ends well! This will be the trip of our dreams; the trip of our lifetime!"

Eric arrives at four this afternoon and he verifies that we have all the necessary documents. He tries very hard to calm me down but unfortunately, with no great success! We go back and fourth to make sure that everything is in order. We check the Frigidaire to verify that what is left will not go bad. During our merry-go-round, Eric places the luggage in the trunk of the car.

And away we go! Eric stops at a restaurant to grab a bite because he knows I do not eat on the plane.

I am beside myself, I cannot swallow a thing but I am very happy! At 6H30 we take off for the airport and we go directly to the first class counter. As the Travel agent said, all is confirmed and the registration is done in minutes. Eric sits with us for a little while and we chat.

We hug and he wishes us a very good trip and most of all to enjoy it to the fullest! After he leaves, we go through customs and shortly after, we board the plane.

XVI

The great reward...

Peter and I are finally in the plane! As soon as the hand luggage is safely stored, we sit down side by side and secure our safety belts. I take Peter's hand and say:
"Darling, I know that I have been a real bunch of nerves and hard to get along with these past two weeks and I am sorry for causing you all that trouble. At this instant I can tell you that we are really and truly on vacation. You know my Love, I was so afraid that something would come up and prevent us from realizing our dream! I was so stressed not to be able to take this plane! Please try to understand Darling. It really was not easy! Now this is our reward: we are both sitting in first class! If only you knew how happy I am, you have no idea... I can assure you that we are going to realize the trip of our dreams. I can even confirm that we are going to make the entire trip, I am sure of it, I can even feel it!"

257

"Sweetheart, not only am I very happy to hear you talk like this, but most of all, I feel revived. I have really been worried about you these past two weeks. You were so nervous, so tense and so scared! I even asked myself if we were going to be able to take this plane. But to hear you talk like this now, I can see that you are feeling better and as you so rightly said: 'Here we are sitting side by side in first class and ready to fly!' I to am convinced that we will have a very good trip! As we promised to one another, let us make this trip the trip of our dreams, the trip of our lifetime! A trip that will hold wonderful memories! It will be such great pleasure to relive them all. If only you knew how happy I am to realize this trip with you!"

Shortly after, the flight attendant comes towards us and offers us a glass of champagne. This time Peter and I stay seated and safely secured to make our toast. We cross arms (like newlyweds) and together say: "To our dream trip and may the Good Lord guide our every step!"

We sip our champagne happy and overwhelmed!

We are sitting in the plane; the motors are rolling; the plane is moving and; it is take-off!

I become white then I turn green! I guess the flight attendant notices my change of color because as soon as she has a chance to get up, she comes towards me.

She offers me another glass of champagne and says:

"Drink it fast; it will help you feel better! You should not worry, everything will be fine!"

She also offers a glass to Peter. I suppose that she thinks he will need it to be able to survive the flight...

I took the pills that the Doctor had prescribed to help calm me. But despite the pills plus the champagne, I still could not sleep a wink!

The flight is calm and seven hours and ten minutes later, we land at the Charles-de-Gaulle Airport.

In Paris, it is 10H30 a.m. on this sunny Tuesday morning, April 27th, 2004!

XVII

Paris...

Finally, we are in Paris; is it possible? I can hardly believe it! We are really here! Dear God, is it really true? This is so wonderful! What accomplishment! What great joy! What a miracle!

Once we pass the customs, we start looking for the shuttle that will drive us to our Hotel. As we come out of the Airport, we see it parked in the said area and the driver is standing in front of it holding a card with the names of two Hotels of which one is ours. There is another passenger with us.

Once we enter the room, we simply drop the luggage and I jump in the mini-bathtub. Peter takes a shower.

We are too excited to sleep, even too tired to try to relax, so Peter and I decide to go for a walk around the Hotel. We want to get to know the surroundings and get acquainted with Paris.

After a few hours of walking and because we have not eaten anything since the little snack on the plane, we pick-up a few sandwiches, two soft drinks and decide to go back to the Hotel. Comfortably installed at the little table in the room we have our lunch and take a little siesta.

We wake up at eight o'clock a.m. the following morning. For a 'little siesta' it was quite a siesta... We go to the dinning room for breakfast and off we go 'en route' for the big adventure.

Shortly after leaving the Hotel it starts to rain, but so little that we hardly notice it. Given that we are living our dream to the fullest and that we are very happy to be here in Paris, it is certainly not a little bit of rain that will stop us from pursuing our constant discovery of this wonderful city. There is so much to see and so little time...

We stop at a kiosk on the sidewalk and buy a few postal cards to send to the children. We continue walking and arrive at a café-terrace and order two bowls of 'Café au lait'. This is so delicious! We sit there and watch the people run all over the place! Rain or no rain, the street is totally crowded!

Simply sitting there is distracting; it must be because we are in Paris! It is absolutely marvelous! I do not know how long we sat there looking all around but all of a sudden the rain stops!

We keep on walking stopping here and there and the first thing we realize, it is already nightfall. We both agree that it might be time to go back to the Hotel.

We have walked all day long and hardly noticed it! I understand now why my feet are so painful…

Our first full day in Paris! The first day of our lifetime dream trip and what a wonderful day it has been! What a great time we had! We are both overwhelmed!

What immense relief to find ourselves here, far from the hospitals, the tests and the treatments. Is it possible to be so happy? Can all this joy be true?

Once we get back to the Hotel, I write a few postcards while Peter takes a good shower. I jump in a warm bath right after.

Peter and I crawl under the nice warm blankets and try to watch a bit of television. It is useless, our eyes become heavy and we both fall asleep. Needless to say that we slept like two contented babies!

On the second day of our journey, we wake up at 9H30. It is incredible! How can we have slept so late? This is not a time to wake up especially when you are in Paris! Peter usually wakes up before six a.m. I guess we both needed this long rest!

After breakfast; back on the road with our little map of Paris and our cameras! We continue the discovery of this beautiful city!

After several miles of walking we arrive at 'L'Arc de Triomphe', built by the French emperor Napoleon at the top of 'Les Champs Elysées' Avenue, in the midst of a huge traffic circle called 'Charles de Gaulle Etoile' where a dozen streets converge.

From 'L'Arc of Triumph' we hop on the most famous avenue: 'Les Champs Elysées' that stretches from 'L'Arc de Triomphe' to 'La Concorde'. At night, it is the most beautiful avenue in the world!

Peter and I stop in the middle of 'Les Champs Elysées' and we kiss. I have never done this before; but I love it!

At this precise moment, I have the impression that we are the only two people on earth! I am lucky to be able to live these wonderful moments with my Sweetheart.

Although my feet are killing me, I just cannot stop; I want to see more and more, so we go on to 'La Place de la Concorde'.

To say the truth, I wonder where all this strength and energy come from! I do not dare question it! I have this strength and this energy and I can only thank the Lord. As we had asked Him, He is watching over us!

At 'La Place de la Concorde', the largest public square in Paris, we see the 'Obelisk of Luxor'. Installed in 1833, it weights 230 tons and stands 75 ft high. It is flanked on both sides by two beautiful fountains called Hittorf, created by the architect of the same name.

We pass through 'Les Jardins des Tuileries' that leads to 'Le Louvre' museum.

We walk and walk and even though Peter's legs and feet are hurting and burning, he is always by my side.

Once in 'Le Louvre' courtyard, we face a huge glass pyramid surrounded by three smaller ones. The pyramids were built by the architect Ieoh Ming Pei. The main pyramid serves as the new entrance to the museum. They provide further lighting and ventilation to the subterranean spaces.

The structure, made entirely with glass segments, has a square base of 115 feet and contains 673 glass panes (603 rhombus-shaped and 70 triangles) but this number was never confirmed. The pyramid was inaugurated by then President François Mitterand.

'Le Louvre' is situated in the heart of Paris. It has been through eight centuries of transformations and expansions thus bringing extraordinary changes in its appearance. 'Le Louvre' is one of the most grandiose and most beautiful art museums in the world.

We find a nice 'balcony terrace' and decide to stop and rest for a while. The arm of the balcony supports at least one dozen of huge statuettes representing an artist, a poet, a king and more.

I admit that a single coffee costs several Euros but to be sitting here at 'Le Louvre' is well worth it. Another part of our dream...

After several hours of walking all around 'Le Louvre' courtyard, we return to 'Les Jardins des Tuileries', the largest and oldest public park in Paris.

This time, we really take our time! 'Les Tuileries' stretches its 'à la française' alleys and beautifully groomed lawns along the Seine River from 'Le Louvre' museum to 'La Concorde' square. The present layout of 'Les Tuileries' follows closely the original layout designed by André Le Nôtre in 1664.

In the center of 'Les Jardins des Tuileries' lies a large octagonal fountain. The fountain is surrounded with chairs where people sit and rest while children amuse themselves. It is relaxing notwithstanding the huge crowd!

After several minutes of rest, we are back on 'Les Champs Elysées'. There are four lanes on each side of the median and the traffic is non-stop.

A little ahead, we see a group of I do not know how many police cars and police officers. Once we get there, they stop several cars and question the drivers...

Peter and I stand there and wonder what is going on! All of a sudden, six police officers surround one car!

First, they question the driver, make him get out of the car, remove the driver's seat and the back seat, open the trunk and the hood of the car and make a thorough search while two police officers watch the driver.

As Peter and I are more and more intrigued, Peter walks towards one police officer to ask him what is going on. All the police officer says is:
"Please move back! Move along!"

The police officer pushes the people back on the sidewalk and keeps on repeating:
"Please move back! Move along!"

After several hours of walking all over, we decide to go back to the Hotel.

In the little street before arriving to the Hotel, we discover several take-out restaurants. We decide to order a nice warm meal and go back to the room. To say the truth, neither one has the strength to go to the restaurant even less to make one step more!

Enough excitement for today! We walked for more than eight hours and we deserve a good rest.

While listening to the news on television tonight, we learn that the police officers of this afternoon were looking for terrorists, weapons and drugs. Finally, now we understand!

We lived another full and wonderful day! Where does all this strength come from? We do not know! One thing for sure; we will start again tomorrow, that is guaranteed!

Fortunately, we wake up earlier this morning! After breakfast, we decide to go back to 'Le Musée du Louvre', the biggest and most beautiful museum in the world. At least, this is my opinion!

We take the guided tour and arrive at 'Les Caryatides' room that owes its name to the four figurines, sculptured by Jean Goujon in 1550. These figurines support the tribune of the musicians.

We continue to 'La Galerie de Michael-Angelo' with its sumptuous marble floor and the well-known painting of the 'Chained Slaves' by Michael-Angelo.

Finally, we arrive in front of 'La *Mona Lisa*' painted by Leonardo di Ser Piero da Vinci at the beginning of the 16th century.

The painting is done on a very thin poplar board and it simply astounds you!

It is the most notorious and reproduced painting in the whole world! While admiring it we understand its worldwide celebrity!

We try to absorb each little detail, for example her expressive face, her eyes that seem to see right through you, her enigmatic smile. Even her arms give the impression she is holding a small child. This painting is absolutely awesome!

We are allowed only seven minutes in front of this masterpiece. Seven minutes is really not long enough to even begin to absorb every little detail of this famous portrait!

Furthermore, when we were there in 2004, 'La Mona Lisa' was temporarily exposed in 'La Grande Galerie' surrounded by several other paintings. The space was too small to contain the huge quantity of visitors.

In March 2005, 'La *Mona Lisa*' was transferred to 'The State Hall' where she has a complete wall to herself. In front of her is the huge painting of 'The Wedding Feast at Cana' by Paolo Celieri (dit Véronèse).

We also visit a few royal apartments including Napoleon III's 'Grand Salon' with all its gold, marble, bronzes, silks, velour and the very rich and ornamented furniture. We must not forget the superbly painted ceiling; it is awesome. Then we enter the Dinning Room; very impressive with its long dinning table and decorated buffet in burnt black wood embellished with gold bronze. The ceiling represents a luminous sky filled with exotic birds painted by Eugène Appert. It is luxurious! What splendor!

We continue our tour through several rooms containing antique Greek and Roman collections, Italian sculptures and statues, frescoes, etc.

At the end of the tour, the one thing that remains in our minds is the picture of 'La *Mona Lisa*'. It is simply the most beautiful painting I have ever seen!

Before leaving Montreal, Peter and I had talked about having a grand outing. We mentioned 'Le Moulin Rouge', 'Le Lido' or even a Diner-cruise on the Seine River. We took pamphlets at the Hotel desk to read on the possibilities. Having read the pamphlets, we still could not make up our minds.

As we walk on 'Les Champs Elysées, we stop in front of 'Le Lido' and inquire at the reception desk. The woman answers several of our questions and hands us a pamphlet saying: "Why not walk down the corridor; you will see several windows offering portions of the show. This will give you a better idea!"

Impressed by what we see, we both decide to reserve tickets for this coming Saturday night. The reservation includes diner and entertainment!

We leave 'Le Lido' both very excited and continue our discovery of this great Paris. As we arrive at the corner of a street; we come face to face with the biggest interior mall; 'Les Galeries Lafayettes'. The place is huge and one can find everything in there!

Coming out of 'Les Galleries', we see several kiosks, all lined up in front of the mall. They have beautiful things and we buy a few souvenirs.

Way too soon, it is nightfall and we must resign ourselves to start back towards the Hotel. The days go by so fast; it is incredible! They are so totally filled that we cannot even see the time fly! At this rate, we will never have enough time to do all that we want...

As we arrive near the Hotel, we stop to buy a few dishes on our little street of goodies! Yesterday's meals were delicious and we are so tired that we decide to repeat tonight. After a delicious meal, we sleep like babies!

What another magnificent day we have lived again today! I know that I will frequently relive all these beautiful moments! I will close my eyes and come right back in this gigantic city filled with history and beauty, including of course the magnificent 'La Mona Lisa'.

We had a very good night's rest and after a good breakfast, we leave the Hotel at 11 o'clock. We had already decided that we wanted to take it easy today!

As we walk, we see a group of buses parked in front of a very big Duty Free Store. Out of curiosity, we decide to go in and see what attracts so many people! We can hardly move in there, it is so crowded!

We do our best to find a sales person because we would like to buy a few perfumes! What a difficult task!

We finally find one and give her the name of the desired perfume. I also ask her to give me some suggestions for a fragrance for Eric. She returns with the required perfume and also hands me four different fragrances to smell. I cannot make up my mind so she asks me to follow her saying:
"We have recently received a new fragrance for an 'Eau de toilette for men' and I hope that it will please you."

As soon as I smell it, I know that it will please Eric. It will suit him perfectly!

As we follow the woman, I see a superb handbag 'Frederica'. I look at Peter and say:

"Sweetie, this would be the perfect gift for my guardian Angel, what do you say?"

"You are right; I think she will really love this bag and appreciate it too."

Once all the shopping is done, we struggle through the growing crowd to get to the cashier. We pay our goodies and are back on the street loaded with boxes and bags.

What a good chance we had finding this sales person, she really was a great help. Whether we bought or not the article required, she always kept her smile and patience and she was very kind to us!

On our way to the Hotel, we see a Wine House and drop in to buy a good bottle of wine for the Oncologist.

They both did so much for me during this terrible and horrific sickness; the least we can do is bring them a little souvenir of our stay in this great city called 'Paris'. After all, it is thanks to my wonderful Doctor who said 'YES' that we are here! We really want them to know that we thought of them during this ecstatic trip. I do hope that our choices will please them both!

Now, we must head back to the Hotel, the parcels are becoming heavier and heavier!

When I think that this morning we left later because we wanted to take it easy! In reality, I think that this day has been the busiest day of all since our arrival in Paris. It was another delightful day!

I am very happy and satisfied with all the nice things that we bought; I am like a child! I am anxious to arrive in the room, open all the bags and examine everything.

Before arriving at our Hotel, we see a Pizzeria and it is mouth watering! I look at Peter and before I can even pronounce one word, he says:
"Darling, would you like to come here for diner tonight? It would be a nice change and besides, it is not too far from the Hotel! What do you say?"
"I guess that you have read my mind; I would love to have diner here tonight! I am really hungry for a French Pizza!"

Once in the room, we throw all the packages on the bed, take a nice worm shower and get ready for diner.

The pizza is baked in the oven, thin crust, with ham, onions and white cheese. We also choose a good bottle of wine to accompany this wonderful meal. A real delight!

After this good meal, we walk towards our favorite terrace and order two bowls of 'Café au lait' that we savor while watching all the people go by.

At 10H30 p.m., we walk back to the Hotel. Once in the room, I examine everything closely! What pleasure to look at each article!

I cannot sleep! I am way too excited with all the good times we have lived here! I hope we will have many more...

272

Tonight is our big outing! I am very excited! Around nine o'clock, we go for breakfast and walk close by.

At two p.m. we decide to take a siesta to be in good shape for this evening.

Awake at 4H30, we get ready and leave the Hotel at 5H30.

Once at 'Le Lido', Peter gives his name, pays and a waiter guides us to our table.

No sooner are we seated, a waiter brings a bottle of vintage champagne and a plate of creamy liver pâté immediately followed by another waiter with a basket of small rolls.

Peter and I are seated face to face at a table of twelve. To my right there are eight Asiatic businessmen and to my left a British couple that complete the table.

There is one bottle of vintage champagne per two people and also a plate of liver pâté. Not only is there one waiter per couple but also another waiter that brings water and serves the champagne and yet another one that clears the table. What grand luxury!

Our table is right in front of the stage and the view is superb! We start talking with the couple to my left and find them very nice.

Slowly the waiters bring the 'entrées'. I chose a Rosette of lobster and its vinaigrette of Sherry and Peter stopped his choice on a fried Foie gras served on a bottom of artichoke in a cream of Sauterne accompanied with a small salad of lettuce sprinkled with walnut oil.

They give us ample time to savor each serving! It is simply exquisite!

After a while they serve a 'Trou Norman': a glass of sorbet with lime and Vodka.

For the main dish, I took: A Filet of beef with shiitakes and its mellow potatoes. Peter went for the crown of lamb roasted in thyme lemon and all its zucchinis.

After giving us a few minutes to digest our wonderful intake, they serve a plate of creamy French cheeses accompanied with a basket of small breads.

For desert, I had a trilogy of frozen chocolate and Peter decided on a macaroon of pistachio and Morello cherry. The meal finishes with a wonderful Liqueur. This was a royal meal concocted by a renowned chef known worldwide.

Throughout the entire meal we have beautiful background music; it is magical!

Towards the end of the meal, the music amplifies and while the waiters clean up the tables, we see a couple of dancers on the dance floor. Needless to say that Peter needed no further invitation to join them.

Believe it or not, on our way back to the table, the Asians next to us stand up, applaud and even give us the 'thumbs-up'!

That was charming and very flattering! Before reaching my seat, I had already grown several centimeters... I too have my little side of vanity!

Can you imagine; two total strangers from a different continent being applauded for their performance? You must admit that it is quite flattering!

I honestly never expected so much and the show has not even started yet!

Once seated, the British woman says: "You dance very well, you give the impression that you are flying. You both have a 'je ne sais quoi' that is very attractive. I wish we could dance like you but unfortunately, my dear husband cannot even keep the rhythm when we dance a 'slow'..."

Suddenly the lights dim, the dancers exit the dance floor and the Master of ceremony appears on the stage.

He welcomes everyone and hopes that we all enjoyed our meal (huge hand of applause). He announces that the show will start in five minutes.

The troupe consists of 60 plus people including: Dancers, Ice Skaters, Acrobats, etc.

Hereafter, I will enumerate the different themes and their acts:
- theme one called: 'The Woman' and it contains eight acts;
- theme two called: 'Paris I love you' with five acts;
- theme three: 'Legendary India', also has five acts;
- theme four and last one: 'Dreaming of stardom'; it too contains eight acts.

The second act of the first theme titled: 'The birds of happiness'; the dancers are all wearing bird costumes.

A lady dressed in a magnificent gold evening gown walks to the center of the stage. While she sings, the dancers fly around her. What a terrific scene!

In the second theme: 'Paris I love you'; the second act: 'Fly to lovely Paris'; all the lights are open and the heads rise to the ceiling. There is a plane hanging from the ceiling; one of the dancers brings a staircase and the dancers start coming down one by one.

I cannot get over the huge quantity of people that come out of that small plane! It is absolutely incredible!

In the last act of the third theme, the spotlights move towards the ceiling of the stage and we see an acrobat coming down. He is suspended with a long white veil around one of his leg. He twists on all sides and discretely, he puts the veil around his wrist. Without a word, he drops several meters at once.

Everyone in the audience screamed; we all thought he had fallen...

The last act of the last theme called: 'Finally, happiness'! All the dancers are on the stage wearing amazing costumes! The men wear royal blue suits, sequined golden vests on a bright white shirt; very elegant. The ladies all have different costumes that are all equally beautiful!

The dances, the singing, the different sceneries, the acrobats, the numerous costumes, all unbelievably beautiful! What a sensation!

If only I could describe each little detail, you.would have so much pleasure to visualize all this beauty! I have never seen anything like it! We are simply flabbergasted!

We must not forget that the dancers change costumes for every scene. I cannot get over it! It is totally awesome!

After the show is finished, there is an unending thunder of applause! Everyone in the hall is standing up and we could hear the 'bravos' coming from all over the place. It is total euphoria!

Before the show, I was already convinced that we would have a wonderful evening but, to say the truth, I never expected so much beauty and such happiness; after all it is the title of the review: 'Le Bonheur'!

For people like us, in the middle class, it was a very expensive outing, but OH, how delicious! This evening was worth every Euro it cost!

We will never regret our decision to come and see this show! It will remain forever engraved in our memories as a dream in color that has come true.

When we finally come out of 'Le Lido', we are still completely ecstatic! We decide to walk for a while; we need to stretch our legs and calm our excitement.

The Avenue of 'Les Champs Elysées' is totally illuminated at night; it is like daytime! What a beautiful Avenue!

The people; they are all over! After all, it is passed midnight and all the terraces are jam-packed.

We finally find a table and order two bowls of 'Café au lait'. We cannot stop reminiscing on what magical night this was!

From this enchanting and magnificent evening amongst other things, we will retain the originality of the costumes and the extravagance of the sceneries.

We cannot stop thinking that no further than a few months ago, I was under the knife for a biopsy, I was undergoing several exams, blood tests and I was receiving 'Rituxan' treatments. Can you imagine?

Further more, once he received the results of the tests, the Specialist tells me that the cancer is in progression and that it is generalizing.

That Peter and I find ourselves sitting at this terrace on 'Les Champs Elysées' in Paris, savoring a nice hot cup of 'Café au lait', after having lived one of the most extraordinary evenings of our lives, is simply incredible! It is surreal!

I understand that such an opportunity is not given to everyone, even less to a 'condemned' person; but as you can very well see, it can happen!

One does not have to go to Paris, nor to 'Le Lido' to realize a dream! Anywhere, anything; as long as it gives you pleasure!

The simple fact of realizing a dream or a project is enough to give anyone the hope, the will to fight, the perseverance, the endurance and the greatest desire to want to live.

Do not ever despair, do not ever let go, fight with all your might, eat well, take plenty of rest, pray and believe in better tomorrows. Miracles do happen and I sincerely believe in them! Am I not the living proof?

Peter looks at his watch and says: "Darling, do you know what time it is? It is passed 2H45 a.m.? I think that it would be a good idea to go to bed!"

Despite the wee hour, neither one of us can sleep! The show keeps rolling in our heads; too much enthusiasm and too much happiness. We cannot stop talking about it!

I have no idea what time it was when we fell asleep; but I spent a long time thanking the Lord for giving me so much.

Tonight my dreams are filled with colors, dances, superb costumes, rich sceneries; including the scenes of a 'Thousand and One Arabian Nights'. Totally fantastic!

I will never say it enough: do not stop fighting, keep the moral high and most of all; never give up. Do not let yourself go to despair! On the contrary, keep the hope and force yourself to smile. Every little effort helps!

The following morning after breakfast, we decide to go back to 'Le Louvre' museum and spend several hours there.

After going all over, we find ourselves back on 'Les Champs Elysées' standing in front of 'Le Lido'. Inevitably, we stroll down the corridor to see the video scenes.

There are still so many beautiful things that we would like to see: 'The Sacred Heart Basilica', 'La Butte à Montmartre', 'The Invalids', 'The Pantheon', 'La Bastille', 'The Notre-Dame Cathedral', 'The Eiffel Tower' and so much more. I honestly do not think that we will have time to see everything!

I simply want to live and appreciate all this beauty that is offered to me so generously. Not only is it very beautiful, it is excellent for my moral! I want to hang on to this precious life with all my strength!

Towards the end of the afternoon, we slowly return to the Hotel. As soon as I enter the room, I through myself on the faucets and run a nice, warm bath. I have an urgent need to soak my poor soar feet and relax in a nice warm bath.

Tonight we eat at the hour of the French society! We found a nice cozy restaurant! The place is totally full and it is already ten p.m.

Another wonderful day! The only complaint that I can think of is that time goes by way too fast. I would like it if this magnificent dream would never end!

Early this morning I call the Travel agency and ask them what would be the price for an upgrade to first class and if there are any seats available. The answer is 'yes' to both my questions and the she gives me the details to get to their offices, in the 12th District, because she has to make the change on the tickets themselves.

We wait until nine a.m. because I want to call Lily at the office. To my great surprise, a night watchman answers. I ask to speak to Lily and he says:
"She has not yet arrived! She only starts work at 8H30 a.m."
"I do not understand! It is three p.m. in Montreal; is she not working today?"
"I am sorry Madam, but it is three a.m. here and she only starts at 8H30 a.m."

I am completely at a loss! I do not understand! I try to calculate the time zone difference.
'There is a difference of six hours between our two continents! Why is it not three p.m.?'

Suddenly I see the light: I reversed the difference! Paris is six hours ahead of Montreal and not six hours behind.

I do not understand how I could have made such an error! I have always known this!

I guess I am too anxious to talk with Lily! It could also be because I am too overwhelmed with this great trip! Whatever the reason, I apologize and say that I will call later!

I tell Peter about the boo-boo I made and we both burst out laughing! We take our tickets and leave for the Travel agency.

This is the first time that we take the metro since we arrived in Paris! While walking towards the agency, I find a Post Office. Finally, I will be able to stamp my postcards and mail them. When we get to the agency, the woman stamps our two tickets and that is it; all is taken care of!

We go back on the metro and get off at the Military School exit because we want to go to the Eiffel Tower. We have never been around here before!

On the other side of the street, there is a beautiful terrace. I am getting quite hungry so we decide to take a snack after which we walk towards the Eiffel Tower.

As we walk, Peter says:
"I am very happy that we had a bite to eat before going up to the top of the Tower."
"Go up to the top of the Tower? Never in your life! Peter, you know very well that I am claustrophobic and I also suffer from vertigo. You will never get me up there, never! I am going to die, I assure you! Oh no, you cannot do this! You must believe me; I am very serious, I cannot do it!"

Believe it or not, he wins! I am shaking like a leaf all the way up, but I go up! I cannot believe it myself! I must admit that from up here, the view is breathtaking!

To see Paris at a glance is really something! The Seine River, the numerous bridges, the boats; everything is miniaturized. It is really something to see! I am very grateful that they have this big wire-like fence all around...

I film everything I see! We stay up there for over an hour!

I must add that it is a beautiful sunny day and Thank God, there is absolutely no wind!

Back down-to-earth, we stretch out on the grass in the beautiful gardens and relax. After a while, we return to the Hotel.

Tonight, we will dine in a beautiful restaurant that we found on the way back.

After a delicious meal, we stop at our preferred terrace for our bowls of 'Café au lait'. Nothing better for a good digestion!

Paris is a nightlife city! The streets are filled with people at all hours! Wherever you find yourself, you find people!

It is a fantastic evening and neither one of us want to go back to the Hotel.

We are so happy and content to be here, far away from the hospitals, the tests and everything else. The one thing that I really miss is the presence of my children and my 'Mine-Mines'.

Peter looks at his watch; it is 2H30 a.m. We think that it is a 'respectable' time to head back to the Hotel! We want to sleep a little; tomorrow is another day!

Only three days left before the next stop!

We could not have planned our trip any better! To this day, everything has been absolutely perfect!

The sky is full of clouds today and it is cold and windy! After breakfast, we go out but we soon realize that we are not sufficiently dressed. We stop at a store and buy two quilted jackets!

The Travel agent had already rented a car for the trip to Germany. Off we go to the car Rental agency near the 'St-Lazar Station' to make sure that all is confirmed and in motion for us to pick-up the car on Friday morning.

Neither cold nor wind will stop us from filling up every single day we have left.

To date, the weather has been nice to us and it is normal to have a gloomy day.

Peter had bought lottery tickets, so we stop at a Cigar Store to verify our numbers.

We discover with pleasure that we have won 36, 80 Euros. It might not be the jackpot, but it is always nice to win! We are very happy and suddenly the temperature does not seem to be so bad!

We continue our walk and take different little streets. All of a sudden, we come face to face with the 'Opera de Paris'. What a nice building with its golden sculptures on its façade! It is huge and simply magnificent! Unfortunately, we cannot visit the interior because it is being renovated.

We walk around and realize that 'Les Galeries Lafayette' are very close by.

After this very long walk, a nice hot mini-bath is a must! As soon as I get out of the mini-bathtub, I jump under the blankets. God, how good it feels to lie down in a nice warm bed! Needless to say that we both sink into lala land very quickly!

We wake up at 8H15 p.m. We dress-up warmly and go out to diner.

As we pass in front of the reception, Peter asks the receptionist if he knows of a seafood restaurant close by. He recommends a well-known place! I love seafood! With no hesitation, we go and enjoy an excellent meal!

Today is already our ninth day in Paris and the first part of our dream trip is nearing the end... We did not even see half of what we wanted to see! We are both completely satisfied and happy of our stay so far!

On our way down to breakfast, unwillingly we hear the receptionist talking to a couple and saying:

"...we have a hail storm since last night! We very seldom have hail here in Paris, especially at this time of year..."

Peter and I look at one another and we can hardly believe what we are hearing! We still have a bit of shopping to do and there is only one day left. We know very well that we cannot afford to lose this day because of the temperature. It is absolutely unthinkable!

We march down for breakfast and return to the room and put on all the warmest clothes that we have because it is cold. We also grab the umbrellas plus all our courage and off we go for the last minute shopping!

Thank God we know exactly what we need to buy! Therefore, everything gets done in a jiffy!

After the shopping, we reward ourselves with two hot cappuccinos.

We are already well into the day and decide to slowly return to the Hotel. I have to start preparing the bags!

I must say that we are not very hungry tonight and we agree to share a club sandwich and two bowls of 'café au lait' in a small restaurant nearby.

I cannot believe that it is our last day in Paris! Time went by so fast! The temperature is still very chilly, but the sun is shinning.

After breakfast, we are in the streets of Paris for more adventures. We want to memorize each little corner!

After an hour or so of walking, we find ourselves back on 'Les Champs Elysées' going from one window to the next. Inevitably, we arrive in front of 'Le Lido'. We cannot go by without walking down the corridor one last time to see the beautiful videos of the review 'Le Bonheur'. To say the truth, we walk down the aisle twice to really immerse ourselves with these wonderful images!

No cold will stop us from sitting at a terrace to drink our cappuccinos. While savoring our coffees, we enjoy watching the non-stop activity all around us.

After an hour or so, we return to the Hotel to complete the suitcases in order to be ready for tomorrow's departure.

As soon as the packing is done, we get ready for our last diner in Paris. We found a great place, unfortunately I cannot remember the name, but we had a wonderful meal.

As we arrive at the corner of the street before our Hotel, Peter sees a cab that looks big enough to hold our entire luggage. He reserves it for 7H30 tomorrow morning.

It is a beautiful night and we do not want this last day to end! We are not sleepy and do not feel like turning in. We never seem to have enough of the nightlife in Paris! Whatever time; day or night, people are everywhere! I wonder; when do people sleep in Paris ...

Even if we are excited for tomorrow's new adventure, we do not want to lose one second of the time left in this wonderful city.

Unfortunately, all good things come to an end and we slowly walk towards the Hotel. We ask the receptionist for a wake-up call at 5H30; only a few hours away...

What a gorgeous time we had here with all the beautiful things we have seen! I have been so happy here and I thank the Good Lord for allowing us to live these great moments!

Tomorrow is another day, a new adventure... Today Dear God I can only cry aloud:
'Thank You so very much!'
from the bottom of my heart for all that You do for me and all that You give me! I am so very grateful to You!

After merely a few hours of sleep, we are both awake way before the wake-up call! At 5H45, Peter and I are sitting in the Lobby and waiting for the Dinning room to open to take our last breakfast in Paris.

After breakfast, Peter goes to the front desk and settles the bill.

The weather is still grey and cloudy outside! Peter joins me in the lobby and we wait for the cab to arrive. At 7H30 a.m. sharp, the cab is here!

Peter helps the cab driver to put all the suitcases in the trunk and off we go to the Rental agency to pick-up the car that we rented for the rest of the trip.

I cannot help thinking that we would have so many more great things to see and visit! Who knows; maybe there will be another time, I hope! I feel very sad at the idea of leaving this wonderful Paris that allowed me to live such fantastic moments!

How right I was when I thought that:
'Coming to Paris with Peter would be very different! I knew that with him I would discover a Paris like I had never seen it before.'

It is exactly what happened! I loved every moment of our stay, even the 'hail'...

When we get to the Rental agency, they inform us that our rented car has not arrived yet. The rented car comes in at 8H20 a.m. and believe it or not, it is a Mercedes! We had requested an economic car with an automatic transmission; I look at the agent and say:

"What do you mean a Mercedes? We rented an economic car; we did not ask for a Mercedes."

"Madam, this is the only automatic transmission car that is available. Does a Mercedes cause you a problem?"

"We are not complaining about the car; it is a great car! We simply do not want to have to pay a surcharge!"

"Madam, I can assure you that there will be absolutely no surcharge! You will find the car parked in the basement; here are the keys and have a good trip!"

I guess we can say that 'luck' was at the Rendez-vous this morning by giving us a bigger car. With all the baggage that we have, it would have been impossible to fit everything in a smaller car.

Furthermore, with the long trip ahead of us; we surely will enjoy the room and comfort!

Peter and I grab the suitcases and bags and go down the basement to meet our Mercedes. It is beautiful and the trunk is huge. We place everything very easily and finally, we are ready to roll...

We sit in the car; buckle our seat belts and Peter looks for the starter. It is nowhere to be found! We have to admit that we have never driven such a car!

When we see an employee of the agency, we ask him to kindly give us a few tips on the functions on the dashboard.

He sits in the driver's seat, puts the key in the ignition and gives us a few pointers. Needless to say that I was all eyes and all ears!

We thank him and at 8H50 a.m., we are on our way to the famous 'Periphery' to take the A1 expressway to exit Paris.

Everything goes well! We find the exit very easily and we are on our way to Germany to spend a few days with Peter's brother and his family.

XVIII

Germany / Hungary / Vienna

Germany ...

As soon as we leave Paris, it is pouring rain! With teary eyes, I look at Peter and say: "You see Darling, Paris is so sad because we are leaving that it is crying! If only you knew how it hurts me to leave 'my' beautiful Paris after having been so happy here!"

On the way, we stop a few times for coffee and to stretch our legs. Overall, the journey goes well despite the rain.

After passing Frankfurt, we call Peter's brother. He wants to know how many more kilometers are left before arriving and how many hours it takes.

As soon as Francis answers, I pass the phone to Peter because I still have not learned the German language.

Peter chats with his brother for a while then tells him that we have just passed Frankfurt; giving him the name of the town, we are in right now.

Francis says:

"You are at approximately six to seven hours away from here! How is the trip going? I hope that you are not having too much trouble finding your way!"

"So far, all is good! I have a great copilot! As soon as we reach Mansfeld, I will call you back. Talk to you later!"

I remember the trip we had made in 1999 when Lily and her family were living in Plailly, close to Paris. At that time, we had spent 10 days with Peter's family and 10 days with Lily, Marc-André and the 'Mine-Mines'.

In 1999, Peter had not seen his brother since 1945 (54 years). When they saw one another on the exact date of Francis' 70th birthday, they both burst into tears and hung on to each other tightly. They were happy; but the emotion was so strong that they could not hold back their tears!

To see two elderly men sob like this; you can imagine the emotion we felt! It was the first time that I saw Peter cry like this since we had been together. To say the truth, everybody was crying! It was simply overwhelming! Two days after this reunion, it was Peter's turn to celebrate his 67th birthday. We were always 'partying' and 'eating'!

Peter was trying his best to integrate me into the conversation, but it was becoming more and more difficult. After an hour or so of torture, I told him:

"Listen Sweetie, take full advantage of this precious time that you have with your brother and his family. There is no need to worry about me! I brought my knitting and I will have my time once we get to Lily's!"

Peter took advantage of his family and enjoyed them to the fullest! After the ten days, we were on our way to Plailly.

I can easily tell you that after ten days of 'near silence' my voice was ready to be heard! When we arrived at Lily's, I could not stop talking... At that time, we really had a wonderful trip!

Now here we are, five years later on our way to see Francis and his family! We arrive a little passed ten o'clock p.m.

All the lights are on! As soon as they see our car turn in the driveway, they come out running ...

What a warm reception! The two brothers embraced and once again, tears are rolling down their cheeks.

His wife, Alice, welcomes me and takes us inside right into the kitchen where I can see the table full of 'goodies'.

At 1H30 a.m., neither Peter nor his brother seem to want to stop talking and I am so bushed! I touch Peter's arm and say:
"Sweetie, I am really tired and I would like to freshen up and go to bed. Could you please go and get the little suitcase that I prepared for our stay; it is on the back seat of the car."

I say 'Gute Natch' to Alice and Francis and run upstairs. What a delightful moment to slide under the blankets!

The bed is super comfortable and covered with a nice thick down. I had no time to say 'OUF' that I was out! I did not even hear Peter when he came to bed!

We hear noise in the kitchen, which is right under the room and it wakes us. Thank God for the noise, it is already 8H40 a.m.!

I want to take a warm shower and undo the baggage; but because it is so late, Peter thinks that we should go down and have breakfast. He says that they have probably been waiting for quite a while already!

There they go again: talk, talk, talk... We could easily call them the 'word machines'. After nearly two hours of listening to them and wondering if they will ever stop talking, I interrupt Peter and say:
"Sweetie, please ask them to excuse me while I go and take a shower and put our stuff in the cupboards."

Peter tells them what I said and they both look at me and say:
"Yes! Yes!"

I come back down about an hour and a half later and believe it or not, they are still sitting around the table talking! A while later, Peter goes and takes a shower!

When he returns, the four of us go for a walk in the neighborhood!

When we get back to the house, Alice goes directly to the kitchen and starts preparing a thick vegetable and noodle soup that she serves with nice fresh homemade bread. Peter had not eaten this soup since his childhood! It was delicious!

At three that afternoon, their children Theresa and Paul arrive and it is time for tea and pastry: cakes, pies, cookies and more. Everything to keep you slime...

To see all this food: I am totally discouraged! I am not used to eating at all times of the day.

At 4H30 p. m. (10H30 a.m. in Montreal), I go to the kitchen and call Eric.

"Hello Sweetie, how are you? We arrived at ten last night and although it rained all day; the journey went quite well!"

"Hi Mom, I am happy to hear your voice and to know that you had a good and safe trip!"

"You will never guess what kind of car we have! It is a Mercedes! The agent from the Rental told us that it was the only automatic transmission available."

"A Mercedes, WOW! That must be super comfortable... How was Paris?"

"Darling, it would take me several days to narrate Paris! Everything was perfect! We have lived the most fantastic ten days of our lives. We filmed and we will give you all the details upon arrival. Have you been to the condominium?"

"So far, I went twice! I watered all the plants like you told me and I also verified that everything was in order."

"Say 'Hello' to Lily, Marc-Andre and the 'Mine-Mines' for us and tell Lily that I will call her tomorrow for Mother's Day. I love you Sweetie! Take good care of yourself and talk to you soon."

"I love you too Mom and I give you a big hug! Say 'Hello' to Peter for me!"

It felt so good talking with Eric even for only a few minutes! Although we are having a wonderful time and living a fantastic trip, I miss my children and grandchildren more and more every day.

While I am on the phone with Eric, Alice, who by the way is an excellent cook and her daughter Theresa start preparing dinner. I cannot help thinking:

'Oh God; not more food!'

Peter and Francis stay in the living room and reminisce. At 10 p.m., I become very tired and I tell Peter:

"Darling, I have go to bed, I am bushed! Please explain and bid them goodnight for me!"

Once in the room, I can hardly wait to jump into bed! I snuggle under the warm down and fall asleep instantly. Tomorrow will be another big day!

Mother's Day and all their children, grandchildren and great grandchildren are coming over! The place will be full to the roof!

We wake up at nine a.m.; this is terrible! We are so comfortable under the big warm down that nothing seems to wake us up. Peter apologizes for being so late but they both say that it is quite normal! After all, we were on the road for over twelve hours!

When we arrive in the kitchen, their son Paul is sipping a coffee! After breakfast, he takes us to his place. They have a beautiful garden and a rock garden that surrounds the elevated patio. They are well established!

After coffee and a few goodies, Paul brings us back to his parent's home. As I enter the kitchen, the table is dressed with pâtés, breads and much more...

I cannot believe this! We just ate! Now we have to eat again. No way, I simply ask for a cup of tea.

After lunch, we go and visit their nephew and his wife.

Believe it or not, the first thing I see when we enter the living room is a table full of cakes, pies, etc. They invite us to sit around the table and 'eat'...

Back to Francis' home at three p.m., the children start arriving one after the other! The house soon fills up! They offer presents to Alice and I even receive a few. Peter and I are very touched by their delicate attention!

While they gather to eat again, I retire in the kitchen and call Lily to wish her a 'Happy Mother's Day'.

Cassandra answers the phone and we are both happy to have a few minutes to talk to one another. She says:
"You know Mamie, this year there will be no Mother's Day celebration with our usual lobster festival! Uncle Eric says that he wants to wait until you come back!"

I can sense some sadness in her little voice. Poor little Darling, I know how much she loves lobster. I tell her:
"Do not be sad Sweetheart; when we come back, we will have a second Mother's Day celebration! That will be fantastic; yes?"
"Well, if that is the way you look at it, I guess that you are right! In the meantime, Happy Mother's Day Mamie and continue enjoying yourselves. I miss you so much and a big hug to you and Peter!"

Afterwards, I talk with Lily. I am so happy to hear her voice! After wishing ourselves a Happy Mother's Day, we chat a while. We are very sad to be so far apart and are both anxious to be together again.

I join the others in the living room! After I do not know how many cups of tea, I tell Peter that I need to lie down for a while, I am still tired. I do not seem to be able to recuperate even though I sleep a lot!

Peter wakes me up at 8H30 p.m. When I join them in the kitchen, they are all sitting around the table and talking... Alice says:
"'Essen! Essen!'"

I cannot get over so much food! I say: "Sweetie, please tell her that I simply would like a soft drink, nothing else!"

Poor Alice, she has a hard time understanding that I do not eat more than that but she gets up immediately and serves me my cold beverage.

The only German word that I know by heart and I know that I will never forget it for as long as I live is 'ESSEN'. Yes, you guessed right, it means EAT! I guarantee that I am never going to forget this word!

This is already our last full day in Germany. Exceptionally this morning, Peter and I are up at six a.m. Even at this early hour, Alice and Francis are already sitting at the table that is filled with goodies.

Around nine a.m. Francis takes us to visit a few stores; I want to buy postal cards and stamps to send home! We could not even find one and come back home empty-handed!

Their granddaughter arrives with her husband and their baby. I wonder if it is Peter or Francis that told her about the cards; she turns around, hops in her car and leaves. When she returns a few minutes later, she comes towards me and hands me a bag with postal cards and stamps.

I run upstairs and write the cards! Once finished and stamped, I join them.

Peter tells me that Jessica offered to post the cards for me on her way home. I thank her!

We want to leave fairly early tomorrow morning; I ask Peter to put the bags in the trunk tonight.

Peter and his brother do not anticipate tomorrow's departure! They know that they will be very sad especially not knowing if they will see one another again.

At least I know that Peter was very happy to spend these few days with his brother.

At 5H30 a.m., Peter and I make the bed and leave the room the way we took it. We join them in the kitchen for our last breakfast. They both look very sad and so does Peter.

After breakfast, I gather our things! Alice hands me a bag with sandwiches and cakes that she prepared for the road.

Peter kisses Alice and turns towards his brother. They both hold on to each other and the tears flow!

When I kiss Alice, I can only repeat 'Danke, Danke'! When the two brothers separate, I kiss and thank Francis. Peter thanks them for their warm hospitality and we leave! The four of us wave until we cannot see one another anymore...

Hungary ...

On the autobahn to Budapest, Peter stops at the first rest area. He needs to gather himself after all these emotions!

He buys two coffees and we talk a while to help him relax. After several minutes, he feels better and we hop in the car and drive on. We pursue our journey to Budapest and everything goes well!

We arrive in Budapest a little passed eight p.m. It is already pitch black outside and we completely forget to reserve a Hotel room before leaving Germany.

We stop at a gas station to fuel up! I can see Peter in the gas station in full conversation with a taxi driver. He comes out, walks towards the car with a huge smile on his face, and says:
"The taxi driver tells me that he knows a nice Hotel not far from here and not too expensive. He offered to take us there! Do not worry Darling, if it is not to our liking, we will simply go elsewhere!"

We follow the cab driver; he turns in a dark narrow road; this of course is nothing to reassure me! I must say that I am not the bravest person on this earth ...

A little further, he turns again and stops in front of a Hotel. Before Peter gets out o the car, I ask him to make sure to visit the room before reserving.

When he returns, he says:
"You will love it Sweetie! It is nice and very clean! On top of it all, there is an inside parking under the Hotel."
"Thank God for that! I was wondering where on earth you could park! Look, the streets are completely full on each side."

The Lobby is spacious and well furnished! Once in the room, Peter was right; it is pretty and very neat!

As I enter the bathroom, I burst out laughing. Peter joins me and I say:
"Look Darling, I think that this bathtub is even smaller than the one we had in Paris!"

I look at Peter and I can see that he is not laughing at all! He is asking himself if he will be able to stand up in there; at least to be able to take a shower.

The worse thing in all this is that there is a seat in the tub that eats up half the tub. There are about ten inches left for the feet.

I put the cloths in the cupboard and take a good hot shower. Even though it is late, we decide to go for a walk.

It is already passed eleven p.m. and we only had the delicious sandwiches that Alice gave us before leaving; we are both hungry!

However, at this late hour, we do not want to go to a restaurant. We decide to stop in a small grocery store and buy a small liver pâté, rolls, cheese and a bottle of wine. This should satisfy our hunger for tonight ...

As soon as we enter the room, we put everything on the table and enjoy our snack!

At 1H30 a.m. we finally think that it is time to go to bed. Despite the long journey, it was a good day!

At 9H30 a.m. we go down to the dinning room for breakfast. It is a buffet-style and the food is delicious!

Here we go with our little city map at the discovery of this new city.

As I go all over filming, Peter follows behind and he is like a child; he stops and talks to everyone. Every time I turn around, he is chatting away with someone new. This is his village, he speaks perfect Hungarian which makes him a very 'happy camper'!

The view is so picturesque! It is breathtaking! On one side of the street you see pastel painted houses all topped with onion-shaped domes. Facing this very beautiful architecture, you find buildings with glass facades: the ancient and the futuristic facing one another. Quite special!

After a while, we stop at a terrace to pause with a cup of coffee and a pastry.

When the waitress comes towards us, I admire her costume which is of the 18th century, the era of Mozart. It consists of a starched white lace bonnet, a flair skirt and a tight-fitted bodice. She also has a starched little white apron tied around her waist. It is very attractive and very neat!

As I want to see the inside of the restaurant, I decide to go to the washroom! I can admire the beautiful paintings, the antic furniture is magnificent and the decoration is refined and exquisite.

I can also hear a gentle music of Mozart in the background. This restaurant offers a very special character! It is not only very stylish and nice, it is also very enticing!

After being soaked in all this historical beauty, we find ourselves right back in the most futuristic scenery.

Right in front of us stands a huge shopping center of three stories high, all covered in glass from top to bottom. What architecture! It is completely opposite to what we have just seen!

For several hours, we go from one boutique to the next just admiring everything after which our feet are begging for a rest. We decide to stop and grab a bite.

After resting for an hour or so, we hop on a tram and go for a long ride.

The last time I was on a tram, I was about five years old. Right now, the tram is made to measure for us because not only are our feet very soar but it also allows us to see other parts of Budapest.

We are staying in Budapest only four days! We surely will not have enough time to see everything and admire different parts of this beautiful city in such a short time.

Peter has often talked to me about the gypsy music and how much he enjoyed listening to it when he was a young boy.

The one thing that has always fascinated Peter about gypsy music is the extraordinary way the musicians have to make their violins 'cry'. He really wants to listen to this music once more.

The next morning after breakfast, Peter stops at the reception desk and asks the clerk if he knows of a place where they play real gypsy music.

The clerk replies:

"I know that there is a very good restaurant with three musicians that only play gypsy music. I hear that this restaurant is well renowned for its food. Their menu is varied and delicious. Would you like me to reserve a table for you tonight?"

"Tonight would be perfect! Could you reserve the table for seven p.m.?"

Once this is settled, we pursue our touring. We decide to go for a stroll along the Danube. On the Right Banc: the Buda side stands the Saint-Mathias Church, Gothic style. It is in this Church that, on the 8th of June 1867, François-Joseph and the empress Elizabeth (better know as 'Sissy') were crowned King and Queen of Hungary. Today's Church was rebuilt in 1896. Not far is the Bastion of the Fishermen. We can also see the Royal Palace in its entire splendor!

The Left Banc of the Danube called Pest is twice the size of Buda. It is dominated by the majestic Parliament, of a neo-Gothic style, built in 1902 by Imre Steindl.

We also see the Chain Bridge that was the first permanent bridge to relate Buda to Pest. It is also one of the longest suspended bridges in Europe.

There are so many beautiful things to see amongst which the Vajdahunyad Castle, built in 1897 during the celebration of the millennium of Hungary; the Opera House, the Place of the Heroes; the Archangel Gabrielle; the Agricultural Museum, the big Synagogue and so much more. Buda and Pest become officially 'one' in 1873.

After this long walk, we decide to pause with a cup of coffee. We arrive on Vaci Street; suddenly Peter stops and says:
"I cannot believe it! I never thought I could remember this place after so many years. My sister used to live on this street when she was working in Budapest. This is incredible!"

As we turn the corner of Vaci Street, we see a lovely little terrace and we order two cups of coffee. While Peter reminisces, I locate a few boutiques and as soon as I finish my coffee, I leave Peter to his thoughts and go gallivanting in the boutiques.

At two p.m., we return to the Hotel to take a small siesta before dinner. At 6H30 p.m., Peter calls the desk and asks for a taxi.

It is a very 'chic' restaurant and the musicians are in tuxedos! The hostess guides us to a table right in front of the musicians. Peter orders a bottle of champagne! He turns to the violinist and tells him:

"I told my Sweetheart that the gypsies have a very special way of making their violins 'cry' by the way they play with the cords. Do you think you could do this for my Love?"

He slips a bill in his hand.

The musicians start playing and we have the net impression that they are playing for us alone. We take several pictures of them and with them and we order our meal.

We sip and savor our well-chilled champagne and let ourselves be rocked by this wonderfully soft music. Peter even sheds a few tears, he is so moved by this music that brings him back to his childhood.

After several hours of enjoying the rhythm of this soft music, Peter asks the waiter to call a cab and we return to the Hotel.

What a wonderful evening, everything was so perfect! We are back at the Hotel at 11H15 p.m. and revive this magical evening.

What marvelous moments we are living since the beginning of this great trip and all this thanks to a 'dream' I had; to my good Doctor who said 'YES' and to God who allows all this by giving me the necessary strength and energy to continue day after day. He watches over our every step!

We are now closing another chapter of our 'dream trip'! It is incredible how time flies! Half of our trip has passed already!

We leave Budapest at 9H30 a.m. and head for Tatabagna. Peter wants to return to Pusztavam, where he was born.

Once there, we visit the Church and the School he went to and continue towards the Street he lived on. Although his house was renovated, he recognized the lot it was on.

What dear memories this brings back to see all the different places he spent his childhood; very emotional! We can even call this a pilgrimage!

We stop at a gas station and Peter asks the owner if he knows of a certain person that lived here several years ago.

To his amazement, someone does know this woman and shows him the house.

Peter goes to the designated house and rings. A man comes out and recognizes Peter.

He opens the gate and they fall into one another's arms. A few moments later, a woman walks towards them intrigued and her husband tells her that this is her cousin Peter whom she has not seen in over 60 years. Dora falls in his arms and they hug and kiss. The 'word machines' are back in motion.

Peter and his cousins do not seem to be able nor do they want to stop talking. They all talk at the same time; I wonder how they can understand one another!

It gives me the impression that they are trying to condense the past 60 years of their separation into a few hours! I am dazed simply listening to them!

After this visit that seems to have been very beneficial for Peter, we head towards our next destination: Vienna.

Before leaving the Budapest Hotel, we thought of reserving a room in Vienna! At least this time we will not have to search for a room once we get there!

Vienna ...

We arrive in Vienna at seven p.m. Once in the room I place our things and we take a good shower. For dinner tonight, we decide to eat in the room! We order a hot meal and some coffee from the Hotel kitchen.

After this wonderful meal, we get under the blankets and try to look at television. Very fast, we are both sound asleep. A well-deserved rest!

This is the first time that we do not walk around the Hotel to get acquainted with the surroundings. After driving such a long distance and a day so filled with emotions, we need a good night's rest!

We get up at 8H50 a.m. and go down for breakfast! It is another buffet-style with a nice variety of foods. It is delicious!

After breakfast, we are off to discover yet another new city! As we come out, we realize that the main Street is right around the corner from the Hotel.

It is on this Street that we find all the boutiques, the restaurants, etc. In other words, we find ourselves on the most active Street of the city. We walk and walk and I film and film! Once again, we find so many interesting things to see!

Around two p.m., I suddenly become extremely tired; to a point where I hang on Peter's arm and say:

"Sweetie, please stop a taxi; I am very tired and I cannot walk back to the Hotel!"

We both wonder what is happening! It has never happened before!

As soon as I enter the room, I hardly have enough strength to reach the bed and slip under the blankets. Before my head touches the pillow, I am out! Did I faint or did I simply fall asleep; I cannot really say; but I am not aware of anything.

Peter wakes me up at 6H30 p.m. saying: "Darling, it is time for dinner!"

I am still so tired and I do not have the strength to get up! I close my eyes and fall right back into lala land...

I wake up at 6H15 the next morning. Fortunately, I feel better! I guess that the accumulation of numerous hours of walking and driving caught up with me!

Apparently, I did not listen to my body that kept telling me that it was getting tired; therefore, it simply made me understand that I needed the rest. This seems to be the only explanation we could think of! One thing for sure; it gave us both a good fright!

We go down for breakfast at 7H30 and believe it or not, we are starved!

After a good and healthy breakfast, we go back to the room and dress up warmly; it is only ten degrees this morning. We return on the main street and try to recuperate some of yesterday's lost time.

311

I wanted to go to Stadt Park to see the Viennese waltz dancers. Because it is so cold, they have not started performing yet. I was so looking forward to it!

As we walk, we realize that everything is closed today. What a catastrophe!

We are both freezing, so we opt to take the tram and go for a tour! At least, this way we will see a little more of Vienna!

We are going to spend most of next week in Munich with my dear friends Lucie and Achim. We stop in a restaurant for coffee and I call them to make sure that there has been no change in the itinerary.

I have not seen Lucie since 1988 when she came to Montreal for a short visit and Achim since 1985 when we left the Ivory Coast. Needless to say that I am very anxious to hug them both and have a good chat!

Achim answers:

"Hello Achim! How are you? How are Lucie and your girls?"

"We are very well thank you! How are you both? Tell me, when will you finally get here? We are waiting for you!"

"We are both very well thank you! We have been in Vienna for a few days already and we are thinking of leaving tomorrow morning after breakfast. I was wondering if you could give me an idea of how long it takes to get to Munich. Are you in Munich or on the off skirts of Munich?"

"Listen my dear Friend, Lucie will behead me if I do not give her the phone immediately! You certainly would not want this; now would you? We are both very anxious to see again! Hold on, here is Lucie and she will give you all the details on how to get here."

"Hello! Hello! I cannot believe that you are so close by! How are you? How are you enjoying the trip so far? I hope that you are both having a lot and fun and living it to the fullest! At what time will you be arriving tomorrow? You are coming, are you not? I hope that you have not changed your mind..."

She simply cannot stop talking and questioning. I must interrupt her.

So I cry:

"Hello! Hello!"

"Oh, I am so sorry! I do not even give you time to answer. You must understand that I am so happy to talk to you! I am really excited! Give me an idea of about what time you plan on being here tomorrow!"

"We are both very well, thank you and we are indeed having a wonderful time! The trip is wonderful! It is very nice to travel this way! Listen Lucie, we will talk longer once we are together! As I was telling Achim, we are planning to leave Vienna tomorrow after breakfast but we have no idea of how long it will take between here and your home. Knowing that you travel a great deal, I thought you could give us a good idea."

"It could take between three and a half to four hours from Vienna and our place. You must not forget, my Dear that we live on the out skirts of the city. Depending on the number of stops that you make and the speed that you drive, you could easily take up to four hours."
"If I go by your speed of driving, I am pretty sure that we will need a good five hours, if not more. If all goes well, we should arrive in the afternoon. I too am very anxious to see you both. I give you, Achim and the girls a big hug and see you tomorrow!"

The desk clerk at the Sissy Hotel in Budapest gave us the name of a famous restaurant for the best 'wiener schnitzels', a Viennese speciality.

He strongly recommended this restaurant and even gave us the directions on how to get there.

Peter and I decide to go and have dinner at this famous restaurant tonight. Warmly dressed, directions in hand, we go searching for the restaurant. Half an hour later, we still have not found it! Discouraged, we stop at a Hotel on the way and ask the desk clerk if this restaurant really exists.

With a smile, she says:
"Yes, it really does exist! As a matter of fact, it is a very renowned restaurant right around the corner. I do not understand that you have not found it! Would you like me to call a taxi and he will drive you to the door?"

The taxi turns right on the next corner, again right on the following Street and stops. The restaurant is right in front of us!

We arrive at the same time as another couple. The man turns the knob of the door: nothing... he knocks: nothing... I see a note in the window, completely on the left side of the door: 'Closed on Sunday'; and of course, the taxi has vanished...

After having looked for this place for so long and to find ourselves in front of a locked door; we are not very happy! There is nothing we can do except return to the Hotel!

We have dinner at the Hotel dinning room! We go back to the room and I prepare the luggage for tomorrow's departure.

Once everything is done and after taking a nice warm shower, we slide under the warm blankets and fall in a very profound sleep.

XIX

Munich, the reunion...

After a very good night's rest and an excellent and healthy breakfast, we pack the suitcases in the trunk of the car and leave the Hotel at nine a.m.

As we arrive near Munich and as understood, I call Lucie to ask her for further directions. She says:

"I think that the easiest way for you would be to go to this given Street and once you get there, you simply call me and I will go and meet you there. It would be too complicated to start explaining all the different little streets to get here. I will be waiting for your call and again, I am very anxious to see you and to finally meet Peter."

Once we arrive at the street in question, I call Lucie. In less than five minutes, we see a car coming on the opposite side and it stops in the middle of the road. The driver gets out and runs towards us!

I recognize her immediately! I soar out of the car like a bullet and run in her direction. We find ourselves in the arms of one another right flat in the middle of the street!

We laugh, we yell, we cry and through all this, we try to talk... Peter gets out of the car and stands in the doorway! He looks at us with a huge smile on his face. He can hardly believe that I can be so deliriously happy!

As we are in the middle of the street, cars are accumulating! Fortunately, we did not hear anyone honking their horns; at least we do not think we did...

After allowing us to live our euphoria for a few minutes, Peter walks towards us and gently makes us realize that we have totally interrupted the traffic!

When finally we gather our spirits, Lucie looks at me and we both burst out laughing. After regaining our self-control, with a smiling face Lucie says:
"I think it would be best to clear the way, because if we do not, we could create a huge traffic jam! Follow me and we will continue this wonderful reunion at home!"

Once in the parking, we start all over again; laughing, crying, screaming, jumping, and all the rest...

Peter cannot take his eyes off me! For him to see me this exuberant, expressive, and so happy, it fills him with joy and he has a smile that passes from ear to the other...

317

Once the three of us are sitting around the table, sipping a nice coffee, Peter says:
"While you were both in the middle of the street laughing and yelling, some people did exactly like me: they got out of their car and simply looked at what was going on. Most of them had a smile on their faces."

I do not have the impression that neither of us will stop talking very soon! We are so happy to be together; it has been so long...

Now it is our turn to want to condense sixteen years of separation into one single evening. We always have a new subject that comes to mind and off we go again!

It is so easy talking with Lucie! It seems like only yesterday we were sipping a hot cup of coffee. I cannot believe that we are here in Munich at my dearest Friend's home! It seems too good to be true!

After a few hours of chatting and chatting, I suddenly realize that I have not seen the other members of her family. I ask her:
"I still have not seen Achim or your two beautiful daughters! Will they soon be here?"
"For the time being Achim is outside of town at a Congress meeting. It was scheduled a long time ago, but we did not want to tell you about it so that you would not be too disappointed. You do understand. "
"Of course I understand Lucie! Tell me, will we at least have a chance to see them before we leave?"

318

"Of course you will! Achim should come back during the day on Wednesday. Besides, the scheduling of this Congress came after we had already made our arrangements! As for the girls; Sophie, the eldest, is studying in London and only comes home during the weekends. As for Olivia, the cadet, she is in her exam period and she went to a friend's house to study. She will be back towards the end of the afternoon. You know, I appreciate having Olivia to myself for a while, it allows a good report between the two of us especially in her teen year."

Now Peter is the one that calls us the 'word machines'. He does not remember having heard me talk non-stop since the first day we met; several, several years ago.

Neither one of us seem to be able to stop talking! Even through lunch, we do not slow down!

I do not recall what time it was when I finally headed up to go to bed the first night; but I do remember that Peter was sleeping very profoundly.

As soon as we get together the next morning, the 'word machines' start all over again bringing back all the wonderful memories. During breakfast, we try to think of everything that has happened to us in the last sixteen years; since we lost contact with one another. After several cups of coffee and several hours of talking, Lucy says:

"Dear Friends, I have tried to organize my itinerary the best way I could so that I would pass the most time possible with you. But unfortunately, I still have a lot of business to take care of and I absolutely must work a few hours today and also tomorrow. I am very sorry, but I really cannot do otherwise! Therefore, I thought that maybe you would like to visit Munich a little bit. I will take you to the train and you can go and see 'Marienplatz'. You absolutely must see this! It is 'the' attraction in Munich. It is unique and very spectacular! I know that you will enjoy yourselves! I hope that you do not mind!"

"Of course we do not mind Dear! I know how busy you are with your Company and that you have several deadlines to meet. We both thank you very much for whatever time you can afford to give us!"

This said, we grab our cameras and off we go to the train station, which is at a five-minute walk from her home. It has been quite a while since I have been on a train...

Once we come out of the train, I stop right in the middle of the steps while people run all around me. I am frozen and incapable of the slightest movement! My eyes look everywhere but my body is numb!

Peter grabs my arm and pulls me before I fall and get stepped on. I cannot stop looking all around! Everything is magnificent! I am flabbergasted! Peter looks at me and says:

"Cookie, what is wrong with you? You cannot simply stand there while everyone runs around you; you will get hurt! Start the camera! Everything is so beautiful!"

"I do not know where to start! There are too many wonderful things: the buildings, the sculptures... My head is spinning!"

"Sweetheart, simply film everything you see! For example; start with the building in front of us; it looks like a Church (but later we learned that it was the first Town Hall building which now contains a toy museum). It is so picturesque with all its different colors! Start at the bottom, go up and then go around the place slowly. Do you see that terrace there Cookie? I will sit right there and you go and film everything you see."

Once back to my 'normal self', I start filming. I read the writings and discover that the original name of the Square was 'Schrannen'. It was renamed 'Marienplatz' (St. Mary's Square) to ask the Virgin Mary to protect them from the cholera epidemic.

The 'Marien Tower' contains the 'Rathaus Glockenspiel', an ornate clock with almost life-sized moving figurines. The clock chimes every day at eleven a.m., noon and five p.m. The Tower is divided in two separate levels. When it starts to play, hordes of tourists gather on the 'Platz' and gaze up at the Carillon.

There is also a column in the centre of the Square called 'Mariensäule' (Mary's column)!

The column is topped with a gilded statue sculpted by Hubert Gerhard in 1590 but it was erected only in 1638.

As I come closer to Peter, he says:
"Look at all the goodies! I ordered German sausages; I have not eaten such good ones since I left Germany. Taste they are succulent! It is understood that I also ordered a glass of German beer. Would you like a sip?"
"Sweetie, you know that I do not like beer! I am sure that German beer will not taste any better! I would like a bite of the sausage!"

I take a bite and it is delicious! Peter orders a portion for me with a coffee.

At five p.m., the Glockenspiel starts to chime! On the first level, we see moving figurines performing the famous 'Schläffertanz' also called 'Cooper's Dance' which was originally performed by Barrel makers in 1517 at the end of the Black Death Plague.

On the second level, you have scenes from medieval jousting knights that re-enact a famous tournament. The show goes on for about ten minutes!

All the figurines are made of wood covered with enameled copper. Very colorful!

Once the show finishes, the place empties at a record speed!

Peter and I decide to stroll around the circle to look at some windows thus avoiding the rush of the crowd. An hour or so later we hop on the train!

We arrive at Lucy's at seven p.m. and she is already waiting for us for dinner! We find ourselves sitting around the table and the 'word machine' is engaged...

I tell her about my amazement when I came out of the train face to face with that immense building. This is when Lucie explains that it was the old Town Hall of Munich. We also tell her about the rapidity in which the place became totally bare after the attraction.

She has a good laugh listening to all our exclamations... Of course, she has been living in Munich for so many years that she has gotten use to all this!

Lucie and I talk until the wee hours of the morning! We cannot stop reminiscing and never get enough of each other's presence. Tonight again, when I enter the room, Peter is way gone in lala land!

Despite the fact that I go to bed very late, I am still up early in the morning. It is as though I do not want to lose one single second of the time I have with Lucie.

This morning is another warm and sunny day! The temperature reaches 29°. We get ready and join Lucie.

She greets us with a nice hot cup of coffee and we all gather around the dining table. She repeatedly thanks us for bringing the sun and the warm weather. I have to admit that since our arrival, it has been effectively very warm and the sun shines every day. She says:

"We have had very cold and gloomy temperature for over one month now! Since you are here, it has been very nice! Given that you brought this beautiful temperature with you, I have taken a big decision: I have decided to keep you here with us..."

Before leaving for 'Marienplatz', Lucie says:
"I will meet you down town towards the end of the afternoon. I want to take you on a tour of the belt of Munich. At least this way, you will get a chance to see more of the city. I have noted the directions on how to get to 'Maximilian Street'. That is where we will meet at 5H30. It is very easy to find; the street is right behind the New Town Hall where you hear the chimes. I am sure that you will have no problems whatsoever! Have a great day and I will see you later!"

We leave the house at ten a.m. and take the train to 'Marienplatz'. To say the truth, we did not have time to see much of the circle because we were too taken by the carillon.

Once on the 'Platz', we visit several boutiques and go around the different kiosks in the circle. We buy a couple of souvenirs to offer as gifts!

At 10H45 a.m. we look for a place on the big terrace so that we can admire the chimes that start at eleven a.m.

As I am getting quite hungry, we order a few German dishes!

After a great meal and watching the carillon, I take Lucy's directions and we walk towards the place where we will meet up with her. The directions are very clear and we find it right away! We return to the 'Platz' and do some shopping while waiting for the five p.m. show. We want to see it again because it will be the last time before we leave!

At 5H15 p.m. we head for 'Maximilian Street and wait for Lucie. When I see her coming, of course she is running as usual! Lucie always runs!

To walk with her is quite an accomplishment! She is very tall and walks very fast! I must hang on to her arm in order to keep up with her! After hugging, she suggests that we go for a drink before going on the tour.

As we walk on 'Maximilian Street', she guides us to a small terrace right in front of the 'National Theatre'. The Theatre is beside the very imposing 'Residenz' (where the monarchy lives). We find a table and order a nice bottle of wine!

While sipping our wine and admiring the surroundings, I tell Lucie:
"I thank you so much for suggesting that we visit 'Marienplatz'! As you said, it is spectacular! It is incredible, the circle was full again today and you could hardly turn around. We also admired several beautiful buildings. What architecture! All the finesse, all the work it involves..."

While we are chatting, Lucie informs us that Achim has returned and that he made dinner reservations at a place called: 'Le Restaurant de la Gare: l'Isarbrau'. She adds: "We will meet him there for dinner at around eight p.m."

Once we finish the wine, off we go for the tour! While Lucy is driving in the enormous traffic, she comments on different places that we see amongst which:

- The 'BMW Headquarters' are located close to 'Olympiapark'. Karl Schwanzer designed the 331 ft. tall four silver vertical cylinders, between 1968 and 1972;
- The 'Friedensenge' (Angel of Peace); a bronze statue commemorating the 25 years of peace following the war of 1870-1871;
- The 'Prinzregententheater' initiated by Ernst von Possart and built as a Festival Hall for the operas of Robert Wagner;
- From far we can see 'The Notre-Dame Cathedral' with its 'Welch' green and bright onion domes;
- The 'Siegestor' (Victory) Gate, designed by Friedrich von Gartner and completed in 1852, is a three-arched triumphal crowned with a bronze statue of Bavaria on a chariot led by four lions. The inscription, by Wilhelm Hausenstein reads: 'dedicated to victory, destroyed by war, reminder of peace'.

Of course, we saw much more but I cannot remember everything...

We must admit that Lucie knows Munich very well! She is an exceptional guide and gives very clear and interesting descriptions of everything we see.

She drives through the streets in an enormous traffic as though there was nothing there. She talks, signals, turns right, signals, turns left... I find it simply incredible to see her drive! It is as though all the cars clear the road when she comes!

I can only congratulate her for her nerves! I know very well that I would be completely incapable of driving in such a heavy traffic. We must not forget all the one-way streets that are everywhere... Puff! Needless to say that I was breathless quite a few times! Oh lala! My poor heart!

After going through the town for nearly two and a half hours, Lucie calls Achim to tell him that we are on our way to the restaurant to join him for dinner.

As we enter the restaurant, I can see Achim sitting at a table! He is sipping a beer and as soon as he sees us, he gets up and runs towards us!

What great joy to see him again after 18 long years! He has not changed at all if not for a few grey hairs...

We hug and walk towards the reserved table. Peter and Achim seem to get along very well. Of course, Peter is totally ecstatic to speak German with him!

For dinner, Achim suggests several 'specialties of the house'. When the different dishes arrive; everybody digs in and we indulge! What a succulent meal!

They also ordered a few one-liter glasses of homemade German beer. Peter does not seem to have enough neither of the food, nor of the beer not even of the conversation! The 'word machines' are going full speed...

We cannot stop talking of our children and emphasize on how proud we are of them! Of course I am unstoppable when it comes to my little 'Mine-Mines', I cannot stop praising them! I guess that for a parent and a grandparent; it is normal to speak so highly of our precious Treasures!

We are so happy to be reunited with Lucie and Achim after so many years! During the conversation, Achim proposes to take us to visit the 'Neuschwanstein Castle' of Ludwig II (Louis II of Bavaria) tomorrow.

He would have liked to take us to the 'Schönbrunn Castle' where Sisi became Empress Consort of Austria by her marriage to Emperor Franz Joseph. But the Castle is closed due to renovations.

I would have loved to visit Sisi's Castle! I would have enjoyed describing it to my little Cassandra because she and I share secret affinities for the beautiful Empress... Who can say, maybe we will have a chance to visit the Castle another time!

We spend several wonderful hours in the company of my long lost friends! It is very nice to rekindle with our past! What great memories we share again tonight!

I met Lucie and Achim in Africa in 1981 when we were stationed there! They both worked in the Ivory Coast at the time. We soon became very close friends. We were even invited to their wedding!

After talking and reminiscing for over three and a half hours, we think that it is time to go home.

Once we get to their place, the two men talk for a while but soon decide to go to bed. Lucie and I continue talking until the wee hours of the morning.

After a few hours of sleep and a healthy breakfast, Achim, Peter and I leave for the 'Neuschwanstein Castle'.

On the way, Achim gives us several details on different buildings and churches. He explains the onion dome roofs that we frequently see in the small towns that we cross. We also admire the beautiful frescos painted on some houses. Really picturesque!

As we go along, I see more and more tall wooden poles painted and nicely decorated. They look like trees without their branches! Intrigued I ask Achim if there is a special meaning to these poles. He says that they are called 'Maypole' or 'Maibaum' (The May tree). He stops the car so we can get a closer look!

As I walk towards the pole, I have a much clearer view! The pole is very high and has several panels on each side. Following my interrogative expression, Achim explains:
"Here in Germany, May 1st is a very special Holiday! The selection of the tree is very important; it must be at least 30 meters high and be bolted upright. The tree is of either maple, hawthorn or birch. The branches and bark are removed and the pole is painted in white and blue stripes (the colors of Bavaria). The 'Maypole' is adorned with a circular wreath and decorated with carved and painted figurines representing worker's trades such as: carpenter, brewer, cobbler, joiner, and many more... When the pole is completely decorated, the villagers transport it to the centre of town. The entire village gathers to celebrate this tradition in a big festival. Before erecting the 'Maypole', the Mayor of the village says a few words and the Reverend blesses the pole. Given that everything is done manually, it requires strength, knowhow and especially precision. Once they judge that the pole is very straight; they drink a wine called: 'Maiwein'. They drink this wine every spring! You can find a 'Maypole' in nearly all the villages and every year there is a fierce competition between the villages to see which 'Maypole' is the highest, the straightest and the most beautifully decorated. I hope that my detailed explanation answers all your questions!"

"Dear Achim, I really could not ask for more! Your explanation is perfectly clear! Now I know what a 'Maypole' is. Thank you!"

We go back to the car and pursue our road to the Castle.

The scenery is beautiful with all the mountains and their summits covered with snow and all the endless green spaces that lay before us are simply magnificent. We have the impression that we are part of a 'Heidi' film. It is really superb!

As we go, we see more and more religious scenes painted on the houses. I look at Achim and ask him:

"Tell me Achim, do these frescos have a special meaning too, or are they simply beautiful decorations on the walls?"

"We are now in 'Oberammergau of Bavaria'. This town is known worldwide for its painted houses and its sculptured woods! These are the traditional characteristics of the area!"

Once we arrive on the site of the Castle, Achim goes and buys the tickets. He informs us that it is very important to buy the tickets before undertaking the climb that lasts 30 minutes. They do not sell them elsewhere!

Achim strongly recommends that we take a ride to go up because the climb is very steep. Without hesitating one second, Peter and I hop on a carriage pulled by two horses and with several others; we are carried through a very dense forest.

The Castle is nestled on the hillside of the 'Bavarian Alps' and Peter and I know very well that we were not sufficiently in shape to climb on foot all this distance to get to the Castle.

The carriage stops a little before reaching the top and we all get down! There is a kiosk of souvenirs and we take advantage of this halt to buy a few things such as postal cards, mouse pads with breathtaking photos of the splendid 'Neuschwanstein Castle".

There is also a restaurant behind the kiosk where the 'daring and courageous climbers' can take a well-deserved rest and have something to eat to regain their strength.

The 'New Swan Stone Palace' (also called: 'Neuschwanstein Castle') is the most notorious of the three castles that Louis II had built.

The concept of this Castle was initiated when the King listened to the music and operas of Robert Wagner.

The Castle stands at 1008 meters high on the rock of 'Pöllatschlucht'. It contains 465 tons of marble and 400,000 bricks. The first stone was placed on September 5th, 1869.

The rooms of the Castle are fitted with hot air central heating system; running water available on every floor and the kitchen has both hot and cold running water and heated cupboards. The King's master suit includes a secret toilet with an automatic flushing system. Telephones are also found on the 3rd and 4th floors of the Castle.

The King used and electric bell system to summon servants and adjutants. His meals did not have to be laboriously carried upstairs but were delivered via a manual lift.

We must admit that in that Era, none of these modern techniques existed. The sad side of this wonderful 'modern' Palace: it does not have an elevator! As a result of this, we had to climb up a flight of spiraling stairs.

As soon as we enter the fairytale Castle, we can feel an overwhelming power of amazement that brings us back to the Era of bygone love affairs, the Troubadours and their love songs. We can easily pretend to be in the epoch of Napoleon and Marie-Antoinette with the big glamorous balls.

The guided tour of the Castle starts with the *Servants' Rooms* on the first upper floor. Five rooms are opened to the public. The 2nd floor, also dedicated to the domestics, was never finished because of the sudden death of the King in 1886.

All the royal apartments are of Roman style, to the exception of the King's room that is of Gothic style.

After climbing **64 steps** in the spiraling staircase (I know, I counted them one by one) and both of us completely bushed and out of breath, we arrive on the 3rd floor and enter the *Lower Hall.* To the West of the Castle is the 'Throne Room' and to the East, you find the 'King's apartments'.

We arrive at the Byzantine *Throne Room* which measures 15 meters high and 20 meters long. The floor consists of two million small stones symbolizing the animals and plants of the world. The glass gem-encrusted chandelier weighs 900 kilos and holds 96 candles. On the wall surrounding the Throne pedestal, there is a painting of the Twelve Apostles. What a striking room! The 'Throne Room' was completed in 1886; the year the King died.

On one side, we see a gallery with pillars covered in Lapis Lazuli offering a breathtaking view of the mountains. On the other; a majestic staircase of white Carare marble at the top of which the gold and ivory throne should have been placed; but it was never installed.

An anteroom takes us to the *Dining Room;* rather small because Ludwig II always preferred to dine alone. On the table, there is a bronze centerpiece mounted on a marble base that is over one-meter high. It portrays 'Sigurd' fighting with the dragon 'Fafnir'.

The *King's Bedroom:* It is there that Ludwig II was arrested on the night of June 11th, 1886. In contrast to the other rooms, it is sumptuously carved in a Neo-Gothic style. The room is covered with rich embroiled draperies and the Monarch's cathedral-like bed is crowned by the most intricate woodcarving.

It took 14 woodcarvers and four and a half years to complete this elaborate oak carving artwork.

We pursue to the *King's Dressing Room*. The main attraction in this room is the ceiling! In contrast to the other ceilings paneled with carved wood, this one is painted with an illusionary scene; through the open roof we see a garden bower with a trellis of vines and look into a blue sky filled with stars and birds. What a sight! It is absolutely magnificent!

The Neo-Gothic style *Oratory* is accessible via a door in the King's bedroom and is for the Monarch's private use only. The murals, stained glass windows and middle picture on the altar feature scenes of the life of the 'holy' King Louis IX of France who was not only Ludwig's patron saint but also the model of the kind of ruler Ludwig II wanted to be.

We move on to the "L" shaped *Salon* through a door in the Dressing Room. Four columns separate the main room from the 'Swan Corner'.

In this room, the swan leitmotif appears on the curtains and coverings made of blue silk and embroidered with swans and lilies. There is also a sculpted life-size majolica swan.

Between the Salon and the Study is the *Grotto* designed for the King by August Dirigl. A secret opening in the ceiling enabled the Monarch to listen to music from the upper floor. It is without saying the most unusual room in the castle!

A glass door opens by sliding into the 'rock' and leads into the *Conservatory Room*.

The main staircase in the north tower leads to the *Upper Hall* on the 4th floor. It ends with a central column in the form of a date palm tree, which spreads upwards in the middle of a blue dome full of stars. I cannot find the words to express the beauty of this image. It is outstanding!

Next to the column stands a white dragon made of limestone. This dragon is known as the 'guardian of the tower'!

Leaving the 'Upper Hall', we go through the Tribune Passage and into the *Singers' Hall*.

This Hall is the gem of gems! Next to the 'Throne Room', this is the most important room in the castle. It occupies the entire 4th floor. The acoustic is exceptional due to the light but strong wood spruce ceiling.

Although suitable for lavish parties, the 'Singers' Hall' was never used during the King's lifetime. The first concerts were held six decades after his death.

The guided tour ends with the *Kitchen* situated on the ground floor. This room has been preserved as it was in Ludwig's days to the exception of the crockery.

Ludwig II of Bavaria was born August 25th, 1845 in Nymphenburg near Munich. He lived only two years in his 'new castle' and died suddenly on June 13th, 1886 in Berg.

Since his death, 1.3 million visitors come here every year. In the summertime, the castle receives more than 6,000 people per day.

After the visit, we catch up with Achim who takes us to a platform from where on one side; we have the most beautiful waterfall. On the other side is the imposing sight of a daring steel bridge hanging at 148 feet above the 'Pollât River Gorge'. The bridge is suspended to the mountains and is called 'Marienbrüke' (Mary's bridge).

'Neuschwanstein' is one of the best-known castles in Germany making Bavaria a prized destination for tourists.

After this wonderful visit, we go to the car and on our way back, we pass a superb turquoise water lake. The lake sits at the foot of the mountains where the melting snow-covered-summits pour its water into the lake. I do not remember the name of this lake but I clearly remember its great beauty!

Once we get back to the house, I prepare the suitcases because we are taking the road to Paris early in the morning.

For our last diner, Lucie and Achim have invited us to a Biergarden.

Before leaving, Achim suggests that we reserve a room near the Airport for tomorrow night. He makes the reservation and adds: "Tomorrow morning I will take you to the Autobahn 8 so that you do not lose too much time turning in circles."

We thank him for his kindness and off we go, with their two daughters, to the outdoor Biergarden. It is such a beautiful evening!

After having finally found a table for six, Lucie and I walk to the 'cafeteria-like' counters. They have a very large variety of grilled meats, pastas and so much more... We make up our own meal!

During this time, Achim and Peter go to the bar in the center of the garden. They order glasses of beer for everyone. We all savor our delicious meal and have a delightful evening. It is so nice to be all reunited!

We finally return to Lucy and Achim's home a little before midnight. Their two daughters bid us 'goodnight' and retire in their respective rooms.

Achim and Peter sit in the living room and chat away while sipping liquor. A short while after, they too decide to call it a night! Lucie and I continue chatting until the wee hours of the morning. We simply want to take advantage of each second left!

To my taste, time goes by excessively fast! I cannot stop thanking her and Achim for their warm welcome and her great availability. I also thank them for everything they did for us during our stay.

Unfortunately, the trip is nearing the end! At five a.m., we are gathered in the dining room over a warm cup of coffee. Lucie and I are teary-eyed and our hearts are very heavy. We embrace and have a hard time letting go! We hope with all our hearts to have the joy of seeing one another again...

At six a.m., we follow Achim who, as promised, brings us to Autobahn 8 in the direction of Salzburg. Once we arrive at the junction, Achim waves and he takes the right side of the road while Peter goes towards the exit for Autobahn 8.

What a marvelous trip we had during these wonderful 26 days; starting with Paris, then Germany, Budapest, Vienna...

In Munich, all the wonderful places we saw thanks to Lucie, the nice visit to the 'Neuschwanstein Castle' and that gorgeous turquoise lake... I must say that we did make our dream trip; the trip of a lifetime!

Peter tries his best to distract me knowing that I am sad to leave my dear friends not knowing if I will ever get the chance to seem them again. Notwithstanding my sadness, we have a nice trip back to Paris and arrive at the Hotel towards the end of the afternoon.

Once in the Hotel room, Peter passes by the washroom and flat stops in the doorway. He yells:
"Sweetie, you have got to come and see this! I cannot believe my own eyes..."

I run to the door asking myself what on earth could have impressed him so much! There it is: a normal size bathtub and not a mini one. What luxury!

We jumped in one after the other and enjoyed it to the fullest! What satisfaction, it was simply divine!

We go out for a quick bite and rush back to the room. We slide under the warm blankets and try to recuperate with a good night of sleep. Needless to say that I do need a good-night's rest!

We have to get up very early tomorrow morning because we must take the car back to the Rental agency by four o'clock. We then have to take the shuttle that will take us to the departure terminal.

I feel so blessed to have had the privilege of living these wonderful days of joy, happiness and real adventure! There are no words to express the immense satisfaction and well-being that this trip has given me!

And more so, I cannot find words that are strong enough to say 'Thank You' to my Dear Lord for allowing us to fully realize this great trip! Praise the Lord!

After all the hours, days, months and years of suffering, waiting for the results of biopsy and exams one after the other, and yes even after all the uncertainties, fears and worries of not seeing the next day... After all this, I have now lived the most wonderful days of my entire life! Enriching, marvelous and totally 'extraordinary'!

All this thanks to a project, thanks to the good Doctor who said 'yes' and also thanks to my dear friend Peter who followed me everywhere without complaining and lived with me this great and marvelous adventure.

In my prayers tonight, I can see my two 'super' wonderful children and my sweet and loving 'Mine-Mines' that I miss so badly, my good friend René-Luc and Peter's son Rich who constantly gave his Father the strength and the courage to go day after day.

I think of the Oncologist, my guardian Angel, the Doctors, technicians and nurses who worked so hard to save my life. I also think of my friends and all those who encouraged me and gave me the will to live...

My most sincere 'THANK YOU', from the bottom of my heart, to every one for all that you did for me. Thanks to all of you, we have lived our dream trip, the trip of our lives!

XX

The return home...

Saturday May 22nd, 2004, here we are comfortably sitting in the plane, still in first class. Despite my terrible fear of flying, I am very happy and impatient to get back home! I am so anxious to see everyone and squeeze them! I miss them so much!

We have lived 26 marvelous and magical days but I have to admit that it makes me ecstatic to come home and find all my dear loved ones.

Because the flight is in the daylight, I find it a lot better than when we flew to Paris at night. This time, I only turned white; I did not go to green...

Approximately 6H30 hours later we land at Mirabel Airport! It is eleven a.m., we are in Montreal and the sun welcomes us back!

As I raise my head before passing through customs, I can see Lily, Marc-André, Karl-David, Eric, Rick and Diane standing there.

After almost one month of absence and even more so in the conditions in which we left for this trip - good for sure, but one must admit, very daring - the rush of adrenalin that I feel when I see all of them there, is incredible... It is as though all the accumulated physical fatigue since the beginning of the trip disappeared instantly.

What a grand reception! Hugs and kisses, we have plenty!

While Lily holds me tight, she says: "Mom, Cassandra wanted to be here to great you, but she has a big exam Monday morning and has to study all weekend to prepare it. She asked me to give you both a big hug and tell you that she is very anxious to see you."

The guys pick up the luggage and we all go to the condominium.

The children bought wine, almond croissants, croissants, chocolate breads, French baguettes, cheeses, pâtés, and much more. We all gather around the table and enjoy all the goodies while doing our utmost best to answer all their numerous questions on the wonderful trip that we made.

Now to find ourselves together, elbow to elbow (eight around a table that usually sits six), in front of all these delicacies, I cannot begin to express the balm that fills my heart, the immense joy and contentment of finally having all my loved ones around me! I am so happy and excited!

The trip was great all the way! I do not have a single regret or one bad word to say about the trip of our dreams. It was truly fantastic all the way!

To hold my loved ones in my arms, to have them here all around me, I could only say that this has no price. Nothing in the whole wide world can equal this happiness!

After several hours of talking about the trip and answering all their questions; at four p.m. they decide to let us rest and all leave at the same time.

I must say that Peter had fallen asleep in his lazy boy! Poor Sweetheart, he is really bushed! Not only because of the trip itself but mostly for having made the flight back with me; it was not really a rest for him...

I too am quite tired, but I honestly do not feel it! Nevertheless, after they leave, I fall into bed like a 'rag'. We both sleep like two contented and very happy children until the following morning.

How nice it is to wake up in our own things! We do not get tired of looking all over; everything seems new! It is as though we have moved into a brand new apartment! It is terrific!

It is understood that because we were in bed at 4H30-yesterday afternoon, we are both awake at four o'clock this morning. More than twelve hours of sleep, I guess we both needed the rest...

344

Because of the jet lag, it is surely going to take us several days to catch up to our normal time. One thing I can assure you is that it was all worth it!

Lily and Eric call this morning to see how we are and if we are more rested! A little later Rick calls and says:

"During my last trip to Florida, I brought back some oranges and grapefruits. I also have several cans of maple syrup for you. When can I deliver all this?"

"Why not come over for pancakes? When you get here, call us and your Father will go down to help you carry all the parcels."

As a matter of fact, their arms were filled with bags and boxes. We have our pancakes and Rick asks more questions on our marvelous trip.

After lunch, I ask Rick to copy the films that I took with the camera on a DVD so that we can play it on the television. After he leaves, we take a small rest!

This evening, we really take it easy! Thanks to our little siesta this afternoon, we are able to hold out until ten p.m. The day flew by like the wind!

The following day, I continue undoing the luggage while Peter goes out to buy the necessary things to make my 'miracle soup'. I have not eaten my soup since we left for the trip and I really want my red blood cells to stay high and healthy.

Peter and I did not take a siesta during the day therefore, at 6H30 p.m. we are both bushed. Finally, we have no choice but to go to bed. Besides, I want to be fresh and rested for my visit with the Oncologist tomorrow morning.

We both wake up at four a.m. and Peter prepares a healthy breakfast! Of course, we have all the time we need to get ready...

I always take a special care when I prepare myself to go to the hospital. I dress up nicely, I do my face and the effect is really incredible.

The secretaries and the nurses (and believe me, I have met quite a few in the past three years of this horrible sickness), are very complementary towards me and tell me with warm smiles:
"Good morning Madame, how are you today? You look so good and you are always smiling. It is nice to see a smiling face in this environment. It is a pleasure to see you again!"
"Thank you so much for your kindness! Your wonderful compliments touch and make me very happy. 'Yes', I am very well thank God! Every day is a new day!"

When we enter the Oncologist's office, my guardian Angel is there also. The Doctor examines me meticulously!

After writing the resume in my dossier, that gets thicker and thicker with each visit, he looks at us smiling and says:

"I guess you will never stop stunning me, Madame! You look very good and in such great shape! The trip seems to have done miracles for you! The examination is good and the blood tests are normal. All in all, I am very satisfied!"

He turns towards Peter and teasingly asks him:

"Tell me Sir; was she reasonable throughout the trip? You can tell me the truth because I know her quite well by now!"

"Honestly Doctor, I have to tell you that I often asked myself which one of us was the sick one, her or I!"

We all burst out laughing! There was no need to say more! The Doctor looks at me and says:

"I will see you again in three months! As usual, should anything occur between now and the next visit, you must not hesitate to call us. Continue taking good care of yourself and the same to you Sir!"

Before leaving his office, we offer him and my guardian Angel the goodies we had brought from Paris. They both look surprised but seem quite happy! We come out of his office both relieved and light-hearted!

We had a very busy day so far and it goes without saying that at seven o'clock this evening, we are both bushed. It is time to slip under the warm blankets and take a very well deserved rest.

This morning we get up a little later; 5H30; what an improvement! After a good breakfast and a few cups of coffee, we go off shopping because Peter has decided to start cooking. He wants to make a big batch of spaghetti sauce and some meatballs.

When we come back from shopping, Eric calls and asks what we are doing. He would like to come over for dinner tonight. I tell him: "Of course Sweetheart; Peter is already in the kitchen cooking! We could have some nice spaghetti with meatballs. How does that sound? Do not eat any for lunch..."

The afternoon flies and Eric arrives at seven p.m. He joins Peter in the kitchen and together they cook the pasta. The three of us gather around the table and savor our meal.

After diner, we look at a few scenes of our trip! We get to 'The Lido' where I take out the brochure of the show titled: 'Le Bonheur!' Eric looks at every picture and finds the costumes and the 'décors' sumptuous. We end up talking about the trip all evening!

Thanks to Eric, tonight we were able to hold out until eleven! The routine is slowly coming back and the normalcy in our life is settling in.

The following morning, we get up at a much more decent time; seven a.m.!

The first Friday after our return from Paris, Rick calls and wants to come over. He claims he has something to show us!

Once he arrives downstairs, he calls and asks us to come down and join him! He is parked right in front of the entrance comfortably sitting in his new convertible. Of course, he takes us out for a ride on the highway. Needless to say that I am the one sitting in the back seat and believe me, I have plenty of wind! Forget the hairdo!

On Saturday, we go and meet Andrée and Renald at the dance Hall. It is wonderful to see them again! Of course, they want to know everything about our wonderful trip and we spend another evening talking 'Paris'. We talk so much that we even forget to dance... We had a great evening!

When we leave the dance Hall, Peter stops at our Bagel store and buys bagels, smoked salmon and cream cheese for our breakfast tomorrow morning. It is such a nice delicacy for us, we simply enjoy it!

We get home a little passed midnight but we do not feel like going to bed!

We put in the cassette and watch portions of our trip. Finally, at two a.m., we think that it is time to get some shut-eye. What a beautiful day this was, super!

Sunday, we simply decide to take the full day to rest. We enjoy our excellent breakfast and simply hang around the house!

The following Thursday, we drive Rick to Ottawa and on the way back, we go and have lunch with Lily.

Before going back to work, Lily gives us the keys to her apartment and asks us to buy a few things for her. After the shopping is done, we go back to her place and wait for them to come home.

When Lily comes home from work, we talk while she prepares diner and Cassandra and Karl-David set the table. In no time at all, diner is served and we gather around the table to enjoy a good meal.

We are very happy to see the 'Mine-Mines' especially Cassandra that we had not seen since our return from Paris. Now it is her turn to ask all sorts of questions on our trip. We spend such good times together. I treasure every second of them!

Once we get back home, I wrap up the gift that we brought back from Budapest for Andrée and Renald; they invited us for diner tomorrow night.

As Andrée and Renald greet us, we offer them the gift, which in reality is their wedding present. We also give them a few souvenirs that we brought from the different places that we visited. They are very happy and thank us warmly!

They had asked us to bring the cassette of our trip and after a succulent diner; we gather in the living room and play the cassette. Of course, we give numerous details as we go along, although an awful lot of scenes are self-explanatory.

After spending several hours gallivanting in Europe with them, we pack up and come home. It is way past one a.m. and we had such a pleasant evening! What a great feeling to relive all those happy moments. Once again, we had a wonderful time.

Sunday morning, we laze around and have breakfast at 12H30 p.m. As we are well rested, we decide to go dancing this afternoon. We are going alone like two 'grown-ups' because Andrée and Renald have other plans for today.

It goes without saying that at ten o'clock tonight, Peter and I are bushed. We look at one another and agree to call it a night...

The following Sunday, Andrée and Renald come over for breakfast. They give us two CDs of beautiful soft music and we eat our pancakes on the balcony and listen to the CDs. It is a nice sunny day!

After they leave, Peter tries out his 'Wok' and prepares a Chinese dish for diner. He bought a Chinese Recipe book in Paris and now he is experimenting!

He concocts several little dishes mainly with vegetables. I must admit that it really tastes great and even more so, it is fantastic for the waistline!

Here we are on Sunday, June 19th, it is Father's Day and Rick has invited us to the restaurant. We are chatting and enjoying a nice meal when all of a sudden, Diane says:

"Congratulations! It has been one year to the day that you came out of the Hospital after your auto graft of the bone marrow!"

How fast time flies! One year already! I honestly did not see the year go by!

For Father's Day and at the same time to celebrate my exit from the Hospital, Rick orders a bottle of champagne and we toast to two great events...

XXI

Happy episodes...

... as of July 2004 ...

Our car is already twelve years old and to date; it has really served us very well despite a few minor problems...

Before leaving for Europe, Peter had two unfortunate incidents and he does not feel very confident and secure any more!

He mentioned his worries to Rick who strongly suggested that we get a new car before something major breaks down and causes a more serious accident.

On Monday, July 5th, Rick picks us up and drives us to this car dealer that he knows. Actually, it is one of his clients!

When we get out of the car, Peter's eyes are attracted to a small hillock and suddenly, they illuminate like a Xmas tree.

The only wish I had expressed was to have a sunroof!

Like a zombie, Peter walks towards the car. As he goes around it, he yells: "Cookie, it has a sunroof!"

At that moment, I knew we had found our 'new car'! We meet the sales representative to discuss the different details and negotiate the price. Once satisfied; we sign!

Thursday, July 8th, Rick picks us up and we return to the dealer. This time, we take possession of our new car!

Another great accomplishment!

We leave the dealer; Peter is at the wheel of our 'new jewel'. We go to Lily's office to show her our new acquisition. After examining it thoroughly, conclusion: the car passes the test and Lily is happy for us!

After leaving Lily, I call the 'Mine-Mines' and ask them to meet us downstairs to see our new car. They both find it very nice and are also happy for us!

Then we go to Eric's office to see what he thinks about it. We all arrive in the parking at the same time and Eric walks towards us and congratulates us for our good choice.

Now we are both happy! All our loved-ones have seen our new car and they all agree with our choice! Two kids showing off their brand new toy!

In the following days, Peter finds all kinds of reasons to go out with the new car. It is good to see him so happy! After all he have been through, he really deserves it!

The following Thursday, I get up and I do not feel well. I take my temperature, and to my surprise, I read 38.6° fever! I spend most of the day in bed!

I notice that I have an ingrown nail on my big left toe and some redness around the big toe of the right foot.

Lily calls and invites us for diner tomorrow night. As I am not feeling well, I tell her that it will depend on how I will be tomorrow and I go back to bed. I wake up at the end of the afternoon; eat a bowl of my 'miracle soup' and go back to bed again. I really feel bad and I am seriously wondering what can be wrong with me this time! I am very worried and totally stressed out!

The following morning I call my guardian Angel and tell her that my fever is still at 38.5°; even though I take analgesics every four hours. She says she will talk to the Oncologist about it and call back as soon as possible. Not even an hour later, she calls saying:

"I met with the Doctor and he would like to have blood tests, a urine sample and also that you pass a lung x ray. He asks that you come to the Hospital as soon as possible. Can you present yourself to the 4th floor this afternoon; the day-Oncologist will see you there."

In no time at all, Peter drives me to the Hospital where I undergo all the required tests. After all is done, we go up to the 4th floor and wait to see the Oncologist.

After several questions, he decides that I should see my Oncologist as soon as next week and not wait for the previously scheduled Rendez-vous of next month.

Peter and I return home disappointed and worried! As soon as I get in the apartment, I jump into bed! A few hours later, I start going to the washroom every fifteen minutes.

It continues like this throughout the night and even this morning. I find that this is absolutely not normal and I really cannot stay like this any longer! Both Peter and I decide that it is best to call the Oncology Ward at the hospital and see if they can give me something to stop this.

The Doctor on duty tells me to drink plenty of water to prevent dehydration and also adds:
"If between now and Monday things are not better, you will have to come back to the Hospital and the Oncologist on duty will prescribe you some antibiotics."

My two big toes are not getting any better either. Because of this whole situation, we spend the weekend at home.

As scheduled by the Oncologist that I saw last week, I meet with my Doctor on Tuesday morning and he says:
"All the exams that you passed are good and nothing appears anywhere."

I tell him about my two big toes and he examines them. He says:

"I have no idea what this could be but I think that you should be seen by a Dermatologist. I can assure you that this has nothing to do with your cancer! As soon as I get the results from the Dermatologist, we will know more. On the other hand, I am very satisfied with the exams and I must tell you that, even if your cancer is incurable, you still have the right to have fever like everybody else. It is most probably a virus of some kind! Try not to worry too much!"

On Monday, July 26th, Peter and I meet with the Dermatologist. As soon as he sees my big toes, he looks at me with a large smile and says:

"Ah, these are simply hematomas! This happens when the nail of the toe is too long; it hits the end of the shoe and the repetition of this movement often causes traumatisms and hemorrhage under the nail. It goes without saying that both your big toe nails are going to fall off; you must not be too surprised! I assure you that they will grow back!"

After giving me his diagnostic, he starts cutting all the lifted part of the nail on the left foot and takes off all he can on the nail of the right foot. Then he says:

"Be reassured, these are only hematomas! This has absolutely nothing to do with your lymphoma. Of this I am very sure! So stop worrying, everything will be fine."

Peter and I go back home with my two bandaged toes and we are both relieved!

At the beginning of August, we pick up the 'Mine-Mines' that come over for a four-day-visit! They are very happy to ride in the 'beautiful new car' as they call it.

The older they get the more we appreciate and love our two little Darlings! We have long and interesting discussions on various subjects! They talk about their little lives, their dreams and their interests. These moments with them are very precious to me! For their young age, they are very open!

We go swimming at least twice a day, sometimes even three times. Darling Peter dreams up delicious meals that we all enjoy together. We must not forget the most important; 'our romantic dinner'! It consists of a beef and shrimp fondue served with rice. There are also three or four different sauces that accompany the fondue. I always serve their favorite juices in wine glasses! Last but not the least; we have delectable deserts that complete a fantastic meal.

We love these two little 'Mine-Mines' so much! They really are our sunshine and the joys of our lives.

It is as though we have just started to enjoy the kids that already the four days have gone by!

Before driving them back home, we stop at the shopping center to shop around and decide to have lunch there. They love to eat at restaurants!

The month of August is the month of all the anniversaries! It starts with my son-in-law's birthday on the 7th, my son's birthday on the 8th, my brother's on the 9th, my daughter and Peter's brother from Germany are both on the 15th and last but not least; my Love's birthday on the 17th. What a month!

'Poor little old me,' I am left all alone in the month of October! Actually, I really cannot complain because not only am I very spoiled but also I am celebrated for over a week. Once Eric takes us out, another time Lily invites us for a wonderful dinner and sometimes, René-Luc invites us all to celebrate my birthday. There is also Rick and Diane that invite us to the restaurant. On the exact date of my birthday, Peter and I celebrate all day!

Even if the initial visit with the Oncologist had been advanced, by the on duty Oncologist because of the fever I had last July, my Doctor kept the original Rendez-vous date that was scheduled for August 17th.

On the scheduled date, Peter and I meet the Oncologist. He examines me and is satisfied. He adds:
"I would like you to pass a lung x ray. You do not need an appointment for this exam; you simply go down to the Radiology Ward and give them the prescription."

Intrigued, I ask him:
"Why are you asking for this lung exam? Has something occurred?"

"No nothing has occurred! On the lung x ray that you passed last March, we had found a spot; but on the July lung x ray, the spot was smaller. You should not worry about this; I simply want to follow-up on it and see where we stand. Do you understand what I am saying? I do not want you to worry!"

Peter and I are surprised! We were not even aware that there had been a spot in the first place. After the visit, we go to the Radiology Ward immediately and I pass the test. I do not want to wait; I am too anxious to get the results!

As soon as we get home, we start celebrating Peter's birthday! Since Peter and I are together, we have always made a point of reserving the exact date of our birthdays for ourselves. Tonight is no exception; even if we had to go to the hospital.

Rick, Lily, Marc-Andre, the 'Mine-Mines' and Eric call Peter and wish him all the best for his birthday.

Now, it is celebration time! For dinner: a filet mignon, giant shrimps, curry rice and a little salad. This great meal is accompanied with a nice chilly bottle of champagne!

For desert, we each have a nice rich and tasty pastry and I serve his with an extra long candle that sparks. I pay special attention in setting the table nicely and place two perfumed candles in the middle. We also have nice soft music in the background!

360

The atmosphere is quite special and we greatly appreciate this private coziness. Overall and despite the fact that we had to go to the hospital, our day of celebration was a total success!

The following day, Rick calls Peter and asks him if he is available for a few days? He has big repairs to do on the box of his truck and he needs his Dad's help.

I continue checking my temperature and so far, nothing has come out! I am still wondering what causes this fever! I stay constantly in touch with my guardian Angel and she tells me to continue taking the analgesics regularly. I try very hard to control the stress and the worrying!

I did not sleep very well last night! I am not used to sleeping alone any more and the bed seems very big! When I get up this morning, I still have a little fever of 37.9°. I had already planned an outing with Andrée; I am not going to let a little fever like this stop me from keeping my engagement.

Therefore, I eat a bowl of 'miracle soup', I continue taking my pills regularly and I take a long siesta to make sure that I am well rested before my outing!

Towards the end of the afternoon, I drive to the shopping center and wait for Andrée. She arrives about fifteen/twenty minutes later than I and we walk around and do a little shopping.

After a few hours of walking and chatting, we go to a nice restaurant and have a good meal. We really have a great time! It is very pleasant and good for my moral!

I come back home at nine o'clock and take my temperature once more. Thank God, tonight it is normal!

Peter returns on Saturday, August 21st and we spend the weekend quietly at home. Of course, Peter is tired but he is very happy for the three days he spent with his son. He says: "Cookie, Rich offers us to go and spend the month of February in Florida, at his trailer. Would you like that? February is such a cold and hard month; why not take him up on his offer and go for a month in the warm sun! What do you say Sweetie?"

"This is a fantastic idea and it is very kind on his part. Of course, it would please me, but Darling, we first have to get the Doctor's permission before we can give Rick an answer. Do you think he can wait until my next visit to the Doctor?"

"Of course he can! Rick is not in that much of a hurry to get the answer."

The following week, Peter goes back and spends another few days with Rick. I know how happy he is to be able to do this for his son and I am very happy for him.

The month of August flies at a ridiculous speed and here we are at the beginning of September.

Towards the middle of September, Peter and I decide to go on a pilgrimage to 'Ste-Anne-de-Beaupré'! I had already been there with my Mother, but it has been so long ago!

I tell Peter that once we get there, I would like to continue to 'Les Éboulements', where my friend Yolande has a crafts boutique and he agrees. I call Yolande and make the necessary arrangements!

Tuesday, September 14th, we leave for St-Anne-de-Beaupré in the morning! We get there around 3H30 and luckily, there is a mass. We go for communion and as I come back to the pew, I see a priest sitting in the back and I walk towards him. I ask him to bless my two rosaries and the cross that Peter offered me for my birthday last October.

After visiting the church, we burn some lampions and say a few prayers after which we are on our way to 'Les Éboulements'. We arrive at 6H15 and Yolande is waiting for us.

It has been quite a while since we last saw one another and she is very happy to find me in such good shape. We toast to good health with a nice chilly rosé and eat.

The following morning, we have breakfast at a restaurant on the sea! It is such a nice warm sunny day!

Yolande gives us a short tour of the surroundings and we go down the steep hill opening on the St-Joseph-de-la-Rive-river. What a stunning view! It is fantastic!

After a few hours of sightseeing, we head back home! We arrive at 5H15! We had a short trip but a very pleasant one! I was so happy to see Yolande after all that time!

I have another visit scheduled with the Oncologist for October 5th. He examines me and says:

"I received the result from your last lung x ray and it is normal! The spot we had seen previously has completely disappeared! I am also satisfied with the exam!"

After he finishes writing his report, I say:

"Doctor, can we still make projects?"

"Where do you want to go this time? Do you want to return to Europe?"

"No Doctor, we just want to get a little sun in Florida. Do you have any objections?"

"How long would it last this time?"

"About one month! Like the Europe trip, we would go by plane and should anything occur, we would take the first flight back."

"When would you leave?"

"It would be for the month of February. What do you say Doctor?"

"How can I object, everything seems to be fine and you will be in very good hands. I know that should anything occur, you would not hesitate to come back. Therefore, I see no problems and I agree! Although, I would like to see you again in December before you leave; is that agreeable to you?"

"No problems Doctor and thank you!"

As soon as we arrive home, I rush on the phone to call Rick and confirm that we accept his offer and plan to leave towards the end of January. We will verify the availability of the plane tickets and call him back with the details once everything is confirmed.

Here I go again, back on the computer to find the best available tickets! A few minutes later, the tickets are reserved. We will leave on January 30th and return on the 20th of February. I call Rick with the details! Now, all we have to do is wait and hope that all goes well until the departure date.

It is already Saturday, October 9th, 2004! It is not simply Andrée's birthday, but also Andrée and Renald's wedding day!

After getting all dolled up, off we go to City Hall for the wedding ceremony! After the ceremony, we all gather at André and Renald's home for a toast.

Like Peter and I, Andrée and Renald met at 'Le Rendez-Vous' dance Hall several years ago and therefore it is quite normal that they would choose that place for their wedding reception. At 5H15, we drive the newlyweds to the dance Hall; it is party time!

All the wedding guests enter the Hall before the newlyweds and we form a guard of honor to greet them. It is so nice to see them hold hands and run through the guard of honor. As soon as they go by, we give them a good hand of applause.

Andrée and Renald had reserved a section of the Hall near the dance floor. They asked that the tables be set in a U-shape and they are sitting in the bottom of the U. It was well thought of because this way, all the guests surround the newlyweds!

We all arrive to the Hall before it opens to the public and make a toast to the newlyweds. They had ordered a special menu for the event! At 6H30, while the dance Hall is filing-up, the waiters serve the meal to the wedding party.

At 8H30, the DJ presents Andrée and Renald to everyone and invites them to open the dance to their preferred waltz.

While the newlyweds walk to the center of the dance-floor, everyone stands up and gives them a huge round of applause. It is so special; we have the impression that it is a huge wedding with a couple of hundred guests...

Andrée is ravishing in her long white-lace strapless dress and Renald is very handsome in his dark suit. After a few turns of waltz, everyone joins them on the dance-floor. It is magical!

Happiness is all over and I feel so privileged to still be around to participate in such a great celebration. Another great blessing of my Dear Lord!

We drive the newlyweds back home at around two a.m. They are very happy and totally satisfied with everything! They are leaving for their honeymoon tomorrow!

I feel feverish when I get up Monday morning. The thermometer shows 38.3° fever and my throat is soar. I must say that I am not surprised because I did yell and sing at Andrée and Renald's wedding.

I spend most of the following two days in bed and Friday morning, given that the fever does not want to leave me, I call my guardian Angel one more time.

After talking with the Oncologist, she calls back saying:
"The Doctor says that all the last tests that you have passed are good, so you should simply continue taking the analgesics. There does not seem to be anything abnormal!"

Lily and Eric call everyday this week; they are worried with this fever that simply does not want to go away. Actually, we are all wondering why this fever is so tenacious! After all, my cancer is incurable... Can this be a recurrence or what? We are all very anguished and on edge!

To celebrate my birthday in style, Eric has invited all the family for dinner on Saturday night. Now with this fever, they are afraid that I might not be well enough to attend my own party. So I make sure to take my medications regularly and rest as much as possible.

When I get up Saturday morning, I do feel a little better! As a present, Peter offers me nice lingerie. He never stops trying to make me feel better and happier!

While Peter and I are having breakfast, the phone rings announcing a florist delivery. I immediately think that it is probably one of the kids or even René-Luc sending me flowers for my birthday.

When Peter opens the door, he comes face to face with Andrée and Renald who have just returned from their honeymoon. I am not dressed, not even combed! Andrée hands me a beautiful bouquet and a nice birthday card. They wish me Happy Birthday and we hug!

We invite them for a cup of coffee but they decline saying that they simply wanted to deliver the flowers and wish me the best. I really appreciated the fact that they took the time to come over in person to offer me their best wishes.

After they leave, I go straight back to bed! I want to rest as much as I can, hoping I will feel better for Eric's dinner party tonight. I get up at around three in the afternoon and Peter and I slowly start preparing.

I still do not feel very strong, but I am a little better than this morning. I hope to be able to get through my anniversary dinner without getting worse.

As I mention to Peter:
"Sweetie, if I do not feel well during the evening, I guess that we will simply have to come back home!"
"Of course Darling and I am sure that they will all understand!"

Exceptionally this year we accepted Eric's invitation to celebrate my birthday on the exact date. He thought it would be best to gather everyone on Saturday night because no one works the following morning therefore, we can stay up later...

We arrive at Eric's at 5H30 and Lily and her family are already there. My super 'Mine-Mines' greet me with a beautiful bouquet of flowers with burgundy and yellow orchids and a huge burgundy sunflower. It is such a nice arrangement and of course, I can get all the kisses and hugs I want today.

Lily and I join Eric in the kitchen while he puts the final touches to this evening's meal. We offer to help him but he simply wants us to sit and chat with him. I find it fantastic to be there! I honestly appreciate these precious moments with them!

When everything is ready, we gather in the living room and Eric serves the bubbly champagne. (Thank God that I did not take any pills today)! Then we savor the delicious meal he prepared for us.

The menu consists of: scampi with a sweet and sour sauce for the entrée; giant and popcorn shrimps served on a nest of rice for the main course and as desert, my favorite: sugar pie. D.E.L.I.C.I.O.U.S...

We leave around midnight! Peter stops to buy bagels and smoked salmon for our special breakfast tomorrow morning.

Is it because I was surrounded by my loved-ones; is it because the analgesics have taken effect? I am honestly unable to say! All I know is that I feel a lot better and stronger this morning.

We get up at nine a.m. and the celebration of my birthday goes on... We savor a great breakfast and wash everything down with a nice and cool bubbly.

For dinner, Peter prepares our 'special anniversary feast' consisting of; filet mignon, giant shrimps, purée potatoes and good veggies. We enjoy a dinner fit for a queen and king. Another super great day!

I have an appointment with the Oncology specialist in mid-December of 2004 and the closer we get to this date, the more Lily, Eric, Peter and I are nervous and anxious. We have to remember that the three last visits of December 2001, 2002, and 2003 only brought bad news. Therefore, it is normal that this visit shakes us all!

When the four of us are all sitting in the office of the Doctor, he takes his time and examines me meticulously. Thank God, all is good; we can all start breathing again, OUF...

Once he gets through writing his report, he asks the usual questions:
"Do you eat well? Do you sleep well? Do you have abnormal sweats? Do you have any pain?"

Questions to which I answer: 'Yes! Yes! No! No!'

After all is done, we leave his office light-hearted and with sunshine in our eyes! Because Lily and Eric are with us, we all go to a restaurant and celebrate the great news.

Now, another Xmas is just around the corner! Peter and I have a tradition with our little 'Mine-Mines'. Ever since they were very young, they come and spend a few days with us to help decorate the Xmas tree. This year is no exception! Although Cassandra is already 13 years old, when I ask if she is too old to come and help us with the tree, she replies:
"Of course we will go Mamie! Besides, if we do not, you will not make a Xmas tree this year and that my sweet Mamie is completely out of the question."

They come and spend the weekend of December 10 and we have a lot of fun decorating the tree. We must not forget our special Saturday night 'romantic diner'! What precious moments God gives me with my little Darlings.

Sunday morning, Lily and Marc-André come over to pick-up the children and Eric arrives a few minutes later. Peter puts on his 'cook apron' and prepares his 'most famous' pancakes.

Once again, Lily and Marc-André have invited us for the Christmas Eve celebration! As goes the tradition, we raise our flutes of sparkling and make a toast of Thanks for all the goodies that come our way…

We all reunite around the beautifully decorated dining table and enjoy the succulent meal they have prepared for us. After the meal is over, 'Mama Clause' sits on the floor near the Xmas tree and we surround her.

Of course, she starts by distributing a gift to each child because they have been waiting for this moment 'so' patiently! What a balm to my heart to see their smiling faces, their shinning eyes and their exclamations when they discover their gift.

The adults too have beautifully wrapped presents to open and like the kids, are also all smiles.

This Xmas Eve is also a very successful evening...

<u>2005</u> ...

For twelve consecutive years, Peter and I have always celebrated the arrival of the New Year at 'Le Rendez-vous'. We reunite with our newlyweds, Andrée and Renald.

We dance and laugh and at midnight, we greet 2005 with a flute of 'chilly champagne'. The evening runs by in a flash as we have so much fun until the wee hours of the morning!

We spend the first month of the year preparing for our trip to Florida. We will be leaving towards the end of the month.

Rick and his girlfriend are spending nearly all the month of January in Florida and Rick offered to take the biggest suitcase down for us; thus leaving us only the carry-on luggage for the flight.

Here we are driving towards Dorval Airport direction: Florida.

Once we arrive at the Fort Lauderdale Airport, Rick and Diane are waiting for us and take us out to diner.

The following morning, Peter and I go to the beach with Diane to see our first sunrise; it is 6H30 a.m. What a beautiful sight looking at this big red ball of fire rising slowly above the level of the sea.

Without one second of hesitation, I run towards the sea and soak my two feet into the freezing salty water. Once I am in up to my knees, I shout:

"Cassandra, Karl-David, look at Mamie with her two feet in the Atlantic! I love you my sweet Darlings!"

No sooner I finish my sentence, I run out of the freezing water! What sweet pleasure...

Now, let the vacation begin; the ocean, the sun, the heat, the walks with bare arms and bare legs. What a dream to be able to go outdoors in shorts and T-shirts, or in a bathing suit, to sip our coffee at six in the morning before leaving for the beach!

Even in Florida, Peter likes to cook! He enjoys making different meals on the BBQ and of course, we take all our meals on the terrace. It is simply divine to do all these things; especially during the month of February!

To top it all off, Rick has a spa on the terrace! We take advantage of it every day! It is very relaxing to be in the nice warm water. Even when it rains, it is a sheer pleasure to hear the raindrops fall on the awning.

We reunite with our old car and it still runs very well!

Having never lived in a trailer park, I really feared the proximity of the neighbors because the lots are so narrow. We are all one against the other!

I must admit that I am truly amazed to see how cozy it is! Even if we have the impression that we are all lined-up like sardines, the funniest thing of it all is that we easily find our privacy.

374

It is already time to pack-up for the return! We cannot get over how fast the time went by! We had twenty-one days of warmth and nice sunshine! We will not be signing the same song when we get back in the 'big' cold...

As we arrive near the Dorval Airport, the pilot announces that it is minus 15°. It is now time to take out the big coats, rubbers, scarves, gloves... It was so nice in the sun!

The flight was not too bad despite some turbulence! Once out of the Customs, we see Eric waiting for us. I am so happy to see him!

A few days after our return, we invite Andrée and Renald for diner. During the meal, Andrée says that they would like to go to a gym to exercise a little. Peter and I think that it is a fantastic idea and we all agree to put Andrée in charge of finding a gym that would be convenient to all of us.

At the scheduled date, Peter and I go for my visit with the specialist.

He exams me closely and after the usual questions says:

"I am really satisfied with the exam and the blood test is also good. So far, everything is going well!"

"I am happy when you are happy! Doctor, Peter and I would like to sign-up to a gym. Would you agree?"

"I have no objections as long as you agree to go slow! I do not want you to start with a marathon on the first day..."

We burst out laughing and I say:
"I get the message Doctor! I will try to be content with 'half a marathon' for the first day! Who knows, I might attain the full marathon on the second or third day..."

At home, I call Andrée:
"Hello to you both! Have you found anything interesting for the gym?"
"Yes, I found one not far from here! Why not come over for a cup of coffee and we will go and see it together!"
"Start the coffee, here we come."

The gym is quite small but very convenient for us! After all, we are no weight lifters; we simply want to exercise a little...

After a few inquiries, the four of us decide to sign-up.

For several years now, Eric always has a lobster feast on Mother's Day. Because Peter and I were in Germany in 2004, Eric preferred to wait for our return. Finally, with everyone's multiple occupations, we never found time to have our feast.

We are all here this year, so Eric invites us to celebrate this Mother's Day event. Lily and her family are there and we meet the parents of Eric's girlfriend.

We start with the traditional champagne toast and all gather around the table! There is an envelope in my plate. I open it and find a beautiful Mother's Day card titled: 'To an irreplaceable Mother'! Eric wrote:

Thank you.......

Thank you   for having been chosen to be my Mother

Thank you   for being who you are

Thank you   for the courage that you show day after day

Thank you   for going to the gym to keep in shape

Thank you   for the lessons of life and the will power that you give us

Thank you   for fighting with such strength and being with me on this Mother's Day

Thank you   for all that I cannot put in words

Mom, I love you; every day my thoughts are with you!

And he signed: ERIC

On the opposite side of the card, he wrote:

We your family; children, grandchildren and future, thank you for your determination, your constant efforts and all your strength that allows us to be reunited today for this great Mother's Day.

It is signed: your family.

377

This is the most beautiful gift I have ever received! I am so moved! If such wonderful words do not give a person the will to fight even more, to persevere and to conquer this sickness at any cost, I honestly do not know what could be more stimulating.

This very special day will remain in my heart for as long as it will continue beating! I will treasure these precious words to my last breath! I am so happy at this instant...

Peter and I have a big project for next summer. We have decided to give our apartment a super makeover!

I must say that it is not as interesting as preparing suitcases for a trip! A lot more strenuous; but what has to be has to be...

We started early on the morning of July 21st and finished the entire apartment on the evening of August 29th.

Oh yes, I was forgetting! In addition to the painting, I sewed curtains for all the windows and patio doors in the condominium plus an envelope for the down on the bed and a skirt around the mattress.

On Saturday, September 4th, we go dancing with Andrée and Renald and they inform us of their up-coming trip to Florida scheduled for next January. They made their Hotel reservations and are very happy about it. I guess we gave them a taste of our last trip!

A few days later, Rick offers us to spend the month of February in his trailer in Florida.

We foresee big changes for the Xmas Holidays this year! To begin with, for Xmas Eve; Eric announces that he will be receiving us for the reception thus giving Lily and Marc-André a well-deserved rest. They have been taking-on this responsibility for several years already!

In December, I get back on the sewing machine. I want to make sure to have plenty of choices for our numerous outings!

I have another appointment with the Oncologist for the middle of December.

When we get to his office, he examines me thoroughly. After noting my dossier, he says: "The blood tests are good and the exam is satisfactory. Your quality of life seems to be quite good and you seem to function very well. Do you eat well? Do you sleep well? Do you have any kind of pain?"

"For the time being, I feel very good and everything is going well! I must tell you that Peter and I painted the entire apartment last summer and I did a lot of sewing. Therefore, when you say that I seem to be functioning well; I guess the answer is 'YES'. I also have something to ask you; we would like to go back to Florida for about five weeks. This time, we would like to drive. I would really like to avoid taking the plane! I hope that you can understand and that this does not interfere with your decision. Would you agree to let us drive to Florida?"

"You know nothing you do or say stuns me anymore! You are a real 'Jack-in-the-box!' Do not change anything; it seems to work very well for you! For your annual follow-up, I will prescribe another abdominal ultrasound and a lung x ray. Stay healthy and have a very good trip! I will see you again next year! A very Happy Holiday Season to both of you and take care."

On the 17th of December, Andrée and Renald come over for our Xmas dinner and of course, the conversation is strictly: Florida!

It is Christmas Eve and Peter and I are ready for the celebration!

Once we are all together at Eric's place, we have our traditional toast! We gather around the nicely decorated table full of goodies and enjoy a great meal!

For this party, Eric and his girlfriend suggested to have a gift exchange. No one knows who had picked whom; it is really anonymous. Eric had asked a colleague at the office to put all our names on individual papers and insert them in a sealed envelope.

After an exquisite meal and once we are all in the living room, let the games begin!

Here is how the exchange turned-out: Lily picked Marc-André; Marc-André had Peter's name; Dominique and her Father exchanged and so did Dominique's Mother and Eric. I offered my gift to Lily and Peter had my name!

We have so much fun! We are like real kids! What a wonderful idea!

Another super great evening surrounded by my loved-ones! Believe me, I store them all! I am so privileged to have the support of such an extraordinary team!

One more big change in our usual plans! For the first time in the last thirteen years that Peter and I have been together, we will not be greeting the 2006 New Year at our favorite dance Hall 'Le Rendez-vous.'

This year, Rick's children are coming over from Switzerland to meet their grandfather! In order to make this a more special event; Rick reserved a two night stay at a great Hotel.

He is really trying his utmost best to make sure that this New Year is going to be a real success! He wants us to be all together in the same room to celebrate the arrival of 2006.

We arrive at the Hotel a little after lunchtime and while we wait for our rooms to be ready, we sit at the piano bar and order a bottle of wine. The pianist plays nice tunes and more and more people gather around to listen to the soft music.

Once we get our room, we shower and dress-up very 'chic'!

At five p.m., we join everyone in the lobby of the Hotel for champagne cocktails and appetizers.

At eight p.m., we are all invited to our pre-reserved tables for the feast!

2006 ...

A few minutes before midnight, the DJ requires everyone on the dance floor with their hats, flutes, streamers, balloons, etc. At midnight, we kiss, hug, and mutually wish one another: Happy New Year 2006!

The evening is at its peak and goes on until the wee hours of the morning. Disco, social dancing, slows, we have all the tempos. Another memorable evening!

After only a few hours of sleep, we meet again in the dinning room for breakfast. After all, it is the Holiday Season, is it not!

In the afternoon, while the kids go skating then for a swim, Peter and I lurk around the numerous boutiques.

Towards the end of the afternoon, Rick invites us to his room for champagne and to view the photos he transferred to his laptop.

Needless to say that shortly after dinner Peter and I excuse ourselves and retire in our room for a good night's rest. We urgently need to sleep!

The festivities of this 2006 New Year were exceptional and really wonderful! What joy to see Peter reunited with all his family for the first time!

On Tuesday, January 3rd, I undo the New Year's suitcases and start preparing the big suitcase that Rick so kindly offered to take to Florida for us.

The first Saturday of the year, we invite Andrée and Renald to celebrate the arrival of this New Year's and to see them before their imminent departure for Florida.

At mid-January, Peter and I go to the Hospital to pass the exams required by the Oncologist. We also take time to go shopping before leaving for the warm weather!

René-Luc and one of his brothers organize a family reunion, for the 21st of January, including the nieces and nephews. They reserved a hall for the occasion.

We were invited and accepted with pleasure! What joy to see them all again! Some of the nieces and nephews are already grand parents. This does not make me feel younger...

I dance my first 'slow' with my grand' son Karl-David; what a special event! I was so happy to still be around and be able to enjoy such a great pleasure, WOW!

I also dance with René-Luc; it has been so long... We started dancing at the age of nine and I think that, it is a little similar to bicycling, you do not forget that!

Before leaving for Florida, I call my guardian Angel to make sure that all my exams are good. She says:
"All the results are good and the Doctor is very happy; so am I! You constantly amaze us! Now you can leave in peace and have a very good trip. Take full advantage of it all and we will see you in three months!"

On January 27th, it is 'D' day; we leave for Florida! It is still dark outside, but the sun will rise soon. When we arrive at the Thousand Islands' Customs, we trigger the alarm of the radioactivity box.

The Customs officer asks us all kinds of questions on our medical situation and other things... I do not react right away! It is only when he tells us to go to the first door that I light-up and yell:
"Ah yes of course, I had completely forgotten: I did pass an ultrasound and also a lung x ray last January 17th."

Unfortunately, it is too late! They examine the car inside and outside. They pass the radioactivity detector everywhere, even on us. We had a good laugh afterwards, but at the time, it was not funny at all!

The first night, we stop at Harrisonburg and the second at Daytona Beach.

Sunday morning 9H39, our next stop is; Pompano Beach. The trip went well and we are very happy to have finally arrived!

The following morning, up at six a.m. and off we go with Diane to the beach.

In the afternoon, we call Andrée and Renald and ask them:
"When are you leaving? Will we have a chance to see one another before your departure?"
"Yes, we were able to keep the room for an extra night! Therefore, we have all day tomorrow to meet."

384

"That is great! What about dinner tomorrow night?"
"That would be terrific!"

Once the four of us are sitting face to face at the restaurant, Andrée says:
"What a funny feeling to find ourselves sitting in a restaurant in Florida!"
"Yes, it is quite special!"

The days go by so fast; we do not even have time to see them! Up at six a.m.; at the beach for the rising sun at 6H30 and back between 11-11H30. We have lunch outside and in the afternoon, either we go visiting, shopping, or for a nice long walk. To top it all, we can relax and enjoy a nice heated spa.

For Valentine's Day, Peter offers me 12 beautiful red roses, a nice heart with diamonds and rubies and a soft teddy bear. For the evening, we go dancing at the 'Irish Pub' in Fort Lauderdale. Even if the dance floor is quite narrow, we have a lot of fun.

On Saturday, February 18th, on our way to the beach, we see several kiosks side by side along the street. We visit them one after the other and I buy a few pairs of earrings for Cassandra and Lily. I also buy myself a beautiful hat with a very wide rim that will protect me from the sun.

We enjoyed ourselves so much that we decide to go back the following day. At one p.m. I become very tired and we go to a restaurant for lunch. Once seated, Peter says:

"To walk like this for hours reminds me of our long walks on the 'Champs Elysées' in Paris..."

As promised, I call the children once a week and cannot stop babbling about the wonderful temperature that we have day after day. I tell them:

"We have even attained 92° this afternoon. Fantastic wouldn't you say?"

They do not find me funny at all because in Montreal, it is -20°...

On Wednesday, February 22nd, Rick calls and says:

"How is the weather at your place? It is nice and hot?"

"Dear Rick, at this moment the thermometer indicates 90°. Is it cold where you are?"

"To the contrary, it is very warm! Come outside?"

I go out and see his truck in front of the trailer. They are both laughing and very happy to have tricked me. They exult!

Once again, the end of the vacation has arrived! It is time to start packing! We want to leave very early tomorrow morning and prevent the heavy traffic.

For our last evening, we go back to the restaurant that Rick and Diane had taken us to because we had enjoyed it so much.

We leave the trailer at 5H30 a.m. and Peter drives up to Rocky Mount where we decide to stop for the night. We take a nice meal and 'good night to all'!

After a good night's rest and a healthy breakfast, we leave the Hotel at eight a.m.! We arrive at the Adirondaks at eight in the evening and stop at a gas station to fill-up and to enjoy a nice hot cup of coffee.

Having heard on the news last night that they were announcing freezing rain for tomorrow, Peter and I decide to continue driving and get home tonight. We absolutely do not want to have to cross the Adirondaks Mountains in a blizzard or an ice storm!

Gathering our courage, we continue our road and arrive at the condominium a little after eleven p.m. I must say that we are both very happy to be home!

Still very tense and wide-awake, we order an all-dressed pizza and have a good snack at two o'clock in the morning. It is delicious!

On Monday, Eric and his girlfriend invite us to the restaurant. We are both very happy to see them! We distribute the little gifts that we brought for them and talk about Florida.

The following Friday, Lily invites us for dinner and we gladly accept. We offer them their presents and they thank us for having thought of them!

During the meal, Lily and Marc-André are very happy to inform us of their new acquisition. They bought a new home! They are ecstatic! They have been dreaming of this since their return from France in 2000. We are both so very happy for them!

The following day, Andrée and Renald come over for dinner.

The first time Renald came over to our place, we gave him a tour of the condominium. When he entered the 'Mine-Mines' room and saw the huge quantities of plush teddy bears, especially the red teddy with the white nose and white paws, he cried out:
"This is the one I want; the red teddy bear!"

During our last trip to Florida, I found a 'little' red teddy bear (the same red as the one I have at home). Therefore, the night they came over for dinner, I gave it to him as a joke! We all had a good laugh, but he did take it home...

What can I say; teddy bears are another one of my passions!

The next morning, Rick and Diane come over for pancakes and they thank us warmly for the bottle of champagne that we left for them before leaving Florida.

This is the 13th of March 2006; another anniversary for my little 'Mine-Mine' Cassandra who is celebrating her 15th birthday. I honestly appreciate being around to enjoy all these special events with my Darlings!

We call Cassandra early this morning but she has already left for school. We leave a message and will call her back tonight.

As soon as she hears our 'two rocky voices' singing Happy Birthday, she bursts out laughing. Nevertheless, she does appreciate the effort...

Three days later, Lily calls all excited and informs us that they have just signed the bill of sale for their new home! She adds that the move will take place only on this coming June ·26th. The whole family is ecstatic and we are all anxious to see them settle into their beautiful new home... What immense joy Peter and I get out of their happiness!

March 20th is Rick's anniversary and he and Diane decide to go on a cruise to celebrate the event. They come over for dinner the following Saturday.

On April 4th, Karl-David celebrates his birthday. He is now 11 years old. Like we did for Cassandra, we call him early in the morning and exercise our 'great' voices on the tune of 'Happy Birthday'!

He too bursts out laughing! But I know in my heart that he is very happy that his Mamie and his Peter thought of calling him on this important day!

On April 5th, it is our friend Renald's turn to add another year to his 'young years'. We decide to go dancing! Renald is touched that we underline this occasion! Whatever the age, I think that we are never too old to enjoy a birthday celebration! ...

Cassandra is already in her third year high and as an extracurricular activity this year, 25 students have been chosen for a two-week-trip to Spain. Can you imagine the great experience this is for a 15 year old?

Saturday April 8th, Lily, Cassandra and Karl-David arrive at ten a.m. Unfortunately, Marc-André is out of town! Eric and his girlfriend come over at the beginning of the afternoon and we all leave to take Cassandra to · the Airport.

I must say that Lily is very nervous and it is quite understandable. After all, it is the first time she sees her daughter leaving alone on a trip overseas!

The trip is very well organized; they have four adults who accompany them. What a fantastic experience!

It is now time to see the Oncologist once again. On April 11th, Peter and I meet with the Doctor. After his exam, he says:
"The exam seems good, there is nothing abnormal. Your blood tests are good and the last tests were negative. Continue doing your usual and take full advantage of life! How was everything in Florida?"
"It was fine! We had very good weather and saw several sun rises! We also walked a great deal and I can assure you; we took full advantage of every day!"
"That is great! I will see you again towards the end of August. In the meantime, should anything happen, do not hesitate to call. Take good care of yourselves!"

We thank him and leave very satisfied with the visit! Once in the car, I call the children and give them the good news.

Mother's Day falls on the 14th of May this year which is also my Mother's birth date. Therefore, this will give us the opportunity of a double celebration.

As usual, we are all invited at Eric's place for our 'lobster feast'. We toast to another Mother's Day with cool bubbly champagne and in my heart, I wish my Mother a very happy birthday.

Before gathering around the dinning table, Cassandra takes Peter and me by the hand and pulls us apart. To myself, I wonder what big secret she wants to confide to us! With her little voice she says:
"I brought a little something from Spain! It is really not much but I thought it might please both of you."

She hands us a little box and when I open it, I find a beautiful rosary. It is a mother-of-pearl rosary!

I cannot take my eyes away from the rosary and I cannot retain my tears. I tell her:
"Oh my sweet Darling, what a wonderful gift this is! You have no idea how precious this is to us! I am so touched and I thank you from the bottom of my heart for having chosen such a great gift for us."

Peter thanks her very warmly and hugs her! This really warms our hearts!

After this little interlude, we all regroup around the table and enjoy our feast. Dear Eric, he cooked enough lobster to feed an army!

We savor our meal with appetite and wash it down with excellent wines. What another beautiful day!

Today is D-Day! Lily and her family are finally moving into their new home. It goes without saying that we are all there to help and are very happy for them!

What joy to still be part of this great world and have the opportunity to share all these precious events in the lives of my dear loved-ones!

On June 30th, Peter and I go to the Airport to greet Rick's daughter and back again on the 4th of July; this time for Rick's son. They must have enjoyed their first visit because they have decided to come back for more...

Peter enjoys spending as much time as possible with them and they in return, love Peter's cooking and are always happy to come over for a meal. We all have a great time in their company!

We have now arrived in the month of all the anniversaries. Receptions right and left, food, food and more food! The weeks go by in a whirl and I take full advantage of every second of every day!

I meet with the Oncologist on August 29th and he is satisfied with the exam. He also adds that the blood tests are good and asks my guardian Angel to schedule the appointments for the usual annual ultrasound and lung tests. My next meeting is set for December.

Here we are; October 16th and today is the day that I turn the page for another wonderful year of life. I accumulate them one by one and I never tire... To the contrary, I adore every instant that is given to me!

Today is my day to be spoiled and celebrated! The phone starts ringing early this morning and does not stop all day. I enjoy every moment of it!

It is already December 5th! I cannot get over how fast time runs by, it is incredible! I do not even see the days... We have another meeting with the Oncologist. As usual, it is the thorough exam and once again, he is content. With his nice smile, he says:
"Everything is good! I must tell you that I am very happy to see how things are going for you. You must continue in this manner and take full advantage of every day! Happy Holiday Seasons to both of you and see you again next year."

We also offer him and my guardian Angel our best wishes! We leave his office relieved and very happy! After all this good news, we are now ready to celebrate with all our dear Darlings.

As the tradition requires, I call the 'Mine-Mines' and ask them if they are still interested in coming over to help us make our Christmas tree this year. They accept with pleasure and tell me that they could come for the weekend of December 15th.

Once again, the Xmas Eve party was to be held at Eric's place. However, I had a little accident in the early hours of Xmas Eve that forces me to get around on crutches. Because Eric's apartment is on the third floor, no elevators, we had to make last minute changes!

After a few phone calls, it was unanimously decided that the Xmas Eve party was going to be held at our place. Eric, Lily and Marc-André bring everything here and we have our usual champagne toast...

After a fantastic meal, we proceed to a gift exchange! This time, we have the possibility to exchange or steal from one another without being allowed to claim our own gift!

You cannot believe all the fun we have! You can hear the 'Ohs and the Ahs' flying! Once every one calms down and 'all the bets are closed', we dig-in and open the famous present we fought so hard for! Another smart formula that creates an incredible ambiance!

What great fun we have again this Xmas! Everything is perfect albeit the fact that I am roaming around in crutches...

When I think that we have celebrated our 5th Christmas since that famous diagnostic of December 27th, 2001, it simply seems so surreal; I cannot get over it...

Look at all the wonderful things we did and all the special events we lived since the Oncologist told us that my cancer was spreading. It is quite difficult to believe!

We have returned from so far... One must admit that this is like recovering from a horrible nightmare. It is a 'miracle'!

After living and enjoying all these precious moments, how can one not believe, how can one not want to fight, how can one not want to put all their energy and willpower in wanting to survive! How can one not pray with all their might!

On the 27th of December 2006, Peter decides to buy a bottle of our preferred champagne! He feels that the fact of still being alive and well is such an important event and such a huge victory that all this needs to be celebrated.

We toast to these wonderful five years and thank God, from the bottom of our hearts for all that He does for us and for all that He gives us so generously!

I end my story on a musical note! Saturday, December 30th, and in spite of the crutches, we decide to go dancing. As for every time that we find ourselves at the dance Hall since the past fourteen years, when the DJ plays our favorite slow tune, my Dear Peter gently touches my shoulder and whispers these magic words to my ear:

"Madame, may I have with dance?"

Conclusion:

What great times I have lived since the beginning of this terrible sickness and thus, in spite of the suffering and the anxiety that we have all gone through!

To say that I once thought that my life was over! Oh, how I fully take advantage of every second the Lord willingly gives me!

This is quite extraordinary when we stop to think about it. One minute I find myself under the scalpel, another I am knocking on St-Peter's door and the next, here I am, walking on 'Les Champs Elysées' in Paris with my dearest friend Peter.

One can say that God acts in mysterious ways sometimes! To this I add: as long as there is breath, there is life, there is hope...

Am I not the living proof? This is what allows me to keep on repeating that we must never give up, never stop fighting with all our might, and even more so, never stop praying and never stop believing.

I reiterate that only God can decide of the fate of everyone! He alone decides where, when and how He will come for us. As long as it is not completely over, we must force ourselves to fight with all our strength and our soul to retrieve every single breath of life possible.

Since that famous day of December 27th 2001, when I was diagnosed with non-Hodgkin Lymphoma, I see the Oncologist only once every three to four months. In comparison to the times when I saw him every two weeks and sometimes even more, this is quite an improvement and a huge victory for my loved ones and me!

As I am always a part of the Protocol of Research, the Oncologist has to send semi-annual reports to keep them informed of my on-going condition.

As far as the Hepatitis specialist is concerned, I continue seeing him but only once a year.

I have just lived five 'super' wonderful years with the people I love most in this world; my dearest ones. Five years to celebrate the anniversaries of my precious 'Mine-Mines' and five years of life with my love, Peter. I have just lived the greatest and most beautiful trip of my life. I have celebrated my fifth Mother's Day, can you imagine! Let us not forget the delicious lobster feasts that I appreciate so! It seems impossible: five years filled with love, joy, happiness, celebrations and life! My Dear God, how great Thy are!

How can I not constantly repeat that, even if the news are terrifying, even if you feel very bad, even if you think that your final hour has arrived; hang on, do not let go, fight, fight and fight some more.

Fight with all you might and force yourself to eat, try to keep busy with things you like to do, think positive and most importantly, do not ever let go!

Do not let this terrible sickness destroy you and do not allow discouragement to take hold of you. Have faith, have hope and pray very hard. Life is terribly precious!

Life is so worth fighting for; if only for one more day, or even one more breath!

I am very happy, I appreciate every rising of every day and I do my utmost best to live each day the Lord gives me to the fullest.

Acknowledgements:

From the bottom of my heart, I wish to thank everyone who have crossed my path, have helped and supported me during this terrible ordeal. Without even just one of my supporters, Peter and I would have never had the chance and possibility to realise our most daring dreams.

Even more so, I am convinced that without all of you, I would not be alive today! Therefore, I would not be able to narrate these different stages of my life.

What magic words can I find to thank my wonderful children, my super great 'Mine-Mines', my love Peter, my dear friend René-Luc, the knowledgeable Doctors, my wonderful guardian Angel, all the personnel and technology of the hospital, my friends, etc.

Do not worry, I am not forgetting my Dear Lord who has followed my every step and has even carried me during the worst moments of this sickness. If there are stronger words than THANK YOU, then I cry them out to You!

To all the nurses who have devoted so much time and energy and who have given me attention, comprehension and encouragements. You held my hand and stayed by my side without even counting the minutes. To each of you, I cry out:

"THANK YOU for having taken such good care of me, for having so much patience with me, for finding the right words to comfort my children in distress and for your terrific words of encouragement towards my dearest Peter who was so worried."

To my guardian Angel with her eternal smile, always ready to be of service. For her patience, her fast response to my numerous SOS calls, her quickness to transmit all the different situations to the Oncology specialist. For taking care of all the 'Rendez-vous' whether it be with my Doctor, with the other Doctors, for the immense quantity of exams, for her constant encouragement and also for always having reassuring and calming words for both Peter and I. To you my dear guardian Angel, from the bottom of my heart I say:

"I sincerely THANK YOU for everything that you have done and are still doing for me. You have played such an important roll in my being here today and for that, I will always be grateful to you!"

To all the Doctors who have constantly been on watch by consulting one another and digging their brains to make sure that they are doing everything possible. For their persistence in searching for the best procedures that will improve my well-being; for their knowledge and expertise, for their precious time, for their constant words of encouragement, for their tremendous patience and numerous caucuses including; 'the burning patient'!

To each of you personally I say:
"THANK YOU! THANK YOU! THANK YOU!
From the bottom of my heart for all that you
have done and are still doing for me. Without
your constant care and attention, I honestly do
not think that I would still be around today...
Of this, I am very sure! May God bless and
protect every one of you!"

Once again, to all I reiterate my deepest
and most sincere THANK YOU for everything!
I am so happy to still be part of this wonderful
world!

If their exists a more powerful and
meaningful word to express my most sincere
THANK YOU for having given me so much,
then I cry it with all my might!

Encouragements:

      To all who are diagnosed with cancer or whatever sickness it may be, we must fight. We must hang on with all our might. We must have hope. Force ourselves to keep our spirits high and think positive even if at times we think that it is totally impossible. We must pray and also and foremost, we must never let go! With such a severe sickness, our food intake is very important and we must make sure to take plenty of rest.

      Every morning when we wake up, we should go to the mirror and force a smile on our face. As much as possible, do anything and everything that pleases us and makes us feel good. Even the smallest little thing helps! This gives us the necessary courage and strength to keep on going. And most of all, never give up; it is so important!

      This is OUR LIFE we are fighting for and we know how precious life is. I am not saying that this is easy, far from that. I am not guaranteeing that this recipe will automatically cure you. My good Lord no, I know how difficult it may be!

      You may think:

'This woman is totally unrealistic! How can she say things like this? Is she not aware that this is completely impossible to realize.'

Believe me it is not impossible to realize; I know because I have been there! It feels like yesterday that the Doctor said:

"Madame, I have bad news for you, we have diagnosed the big 'C'."

Yes, it feels like yesterday and yet, it was in December 2001. I do know what I am talking about. I know how terrible and difficult it is for the nerves, extremely hard for the body and dreadfully hard for the moral. Difficult and hard yes but, believe me, not impossible!

I can only say that every little bit helps. We must take one step at a time! With time, we will achieve giant steps and we will feel so proud. We must do our utmost to put all the chances on our side!

We should take advantage of every little joy that comes our way! I can assure you that, down the line, they amass and they really help.

I am fully aware that we do not all pull through these terrible sicknesses! I am also aware that the smallest to the biggest effort that we make, we help ourselves and it is so very important. Let it be a simple smile, it makes us feel good inside and it does make a huge difference.

Cancer is very terrifying; it scares everyone. It is like receiving a death sentence. How often have we said or even thought to ourselves:

"Ah! This only happens to others!"

I know, I have often thought it myself! However, when WE are diagnosed; it is completely different! We cannot just stay there and wait for the worst to happen. To the contrary, we must fight to the utmost!

To do this, we must start by helping ourselves! We must fight as hard as we possibly can. We must hang on to anything and everything positive and good for us. Then, only then, will we better benefit from all the help the doctors, the nurses and all our surrounding can give us.

Please, we must never forget, we are fighting for OUR LIFE; we must never let ourselves go to discouragement. As long as there is a breath, there is life, there is hope! We must believe in this! It is absolutely necessary to believe that we will pull through this.

Let us have the satisfaction of being able to say:
'I really did all I could to pull through this awful sickness. I have put all my strength, my energy and my good will into it. Not one doctor, one nurse, not even one person could say, or even think, that I did not do my utmost best. For me, this is a huge victory!'

I do hope that by writing my experience, it will help sick people, give them hope, help keep their spirits high, encourage them to constantly fight with all their might.

My most sincere wish is to encourage you to constantly fight and pray. You must never let go!

To all who suffer, I would like to bring; my faith, my strength, my courage and I pray the good Lord that it could help. Even if I only reach a few of you, then all my efforts will not have been in vain. It will all have been worth it!

TABLE OF CONTENTS